THE COMPLETE BOOK OF HOME HERBAL REMEDIES

THE
COMPLETE BOOK
OF HOME
HERBAL REMEDIES

A holistic guide to understanding and treating

common ailments with herbs

JADE BRITTON
& TAMARA KIRCHER

FIREFLY BOOKS

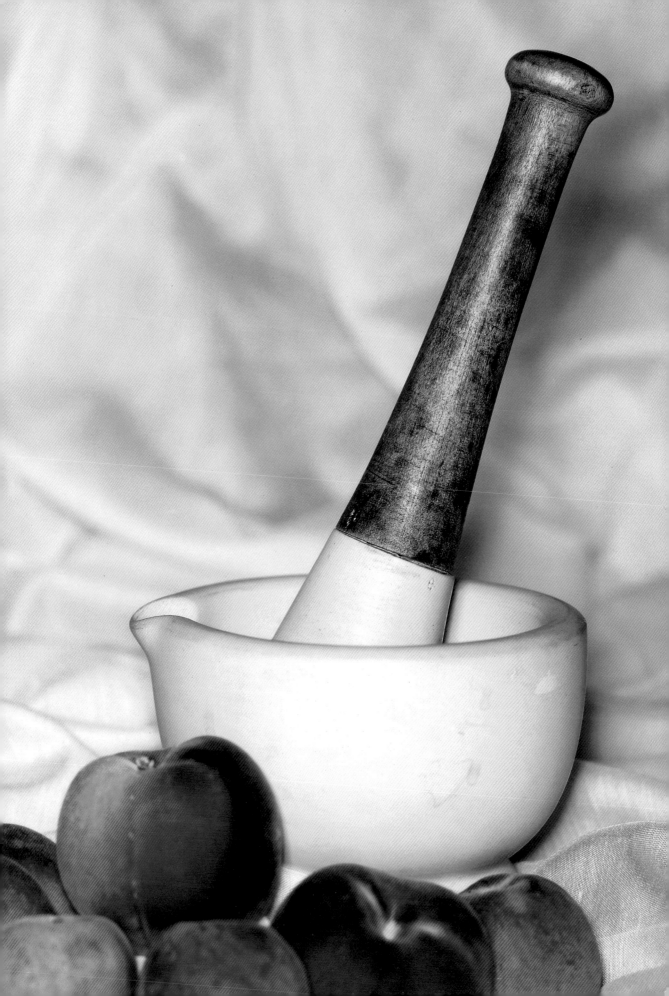

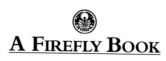

A FIREFLY BOOK

Published in Canada in 1998 by
Firefly Books Ltd.
3680 Victoria Park Avenue
Willowdale, Ontario M2H 3KI

Published in the United States in 1998 by
Firefly Books (U.S.) Inc.
P.O. Box 1338, Ellicott Station
Buffalo, New York 14205

Cataloguing in Publication Data

Kircher, Tamara
Complete book of home herbal remedies
Includes index.
ISBN 1 – 55209 – 176 – 7
1. Herbs – Therapeutic use – Popular works. I. Britton,
Jade, 1956 – . II. Title.
RM666.H33K57 1997 615'.321 C97 – 931653 – 7

This book was designed and produced by
Quarto Publishing plc
The Old Brewery
6 Blundell Street
London N7 9BH

Typeset in Great Britain by
Central Southern Typesetters, Eastbourne
Manufactured in Singapore by
Bright Arts (Singapore) Pte. Ltd.
Printed in China by
Leefung-Asco Printers Ltd.

CONTENTS

FOREWORD 6

INTRODUCTION 8

THINKING HOLISTICALLY 10

HOW TO USE THIS BOOK 13

HERBAL METHODS 14

Infusions 17

Decoctions 18

Tinctures 19

Medicinal Wines 20

Gargles and
  Mouthwashes 21

Eyewashes 22

Baths 23

Inhalations 24

Infused Oils 25

Ointments 26

Creams 27

Syrups 28

Vinegars 29

Poultices and
  Compresses 30

Pessaries and Suppositories 31

Chinese Herbal Decoctions 32

Chinese Patent Formulas 33

THE BODY & HOW TO TREAT IT 36

Healing Herbs 38

Respiration 40

The Eyes and Ears 46

The Digestive System 48

The Urinary System 54

The Reproductive System 58

The Endocrine System 66

The Skin 70

The Circulatory System 76

The Musculoskeletal System 84

The Nervous System 88

The Immune System 96

THE HERBAL DIRECTORY 100

Achillea millefolium to
  Zingiber officinale 102–151

ADDITIONAL HERBS 152

KITCHEN REMEDIES 154

A FAMILY REMEDY CHEST 155

GLOSSARY 156

FURTHER READING AND
  USEFUL ADDRESSES 157

INDEX 158

CREDITS 160

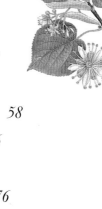

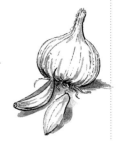

FOREWORD

We are living in a time of great diversity, change, and confusion. We are overwhelmed with choices of healing systems, concepts, and treatment techniques. Some feel that herbal medicine is just one of a variety of alternative therapies. It is far from that, since it is used by up to 80 per cent of the world's population for their health care needs. Herbal medicine does not oppose conventional medicine, but can be used as first line therapy in a more natural healing fashion. In fact, many of today's modern or "miracle" drugs have grown from the roots of herbalism. Even though modern medicine has its basis in herbalism, often a drug is over-refined and may lose some of the other components that complement or prevent side effects.

Plant medicine has been used in a therapeutic fashion since antiquity in the healing of body, mind, and spirit. This philosophy is our heritage. Herbal medicine uses a holistic

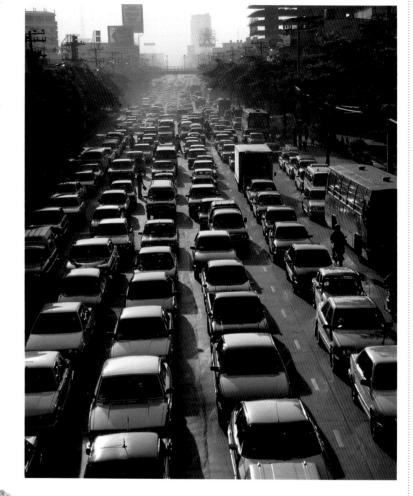

approach to healing and shows ways of life enhancement, rather than just

Pollution caused by our consumer-driven society is threatening our health and the health of the planet as a whole.

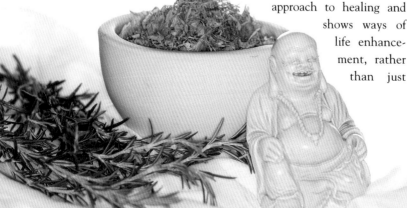

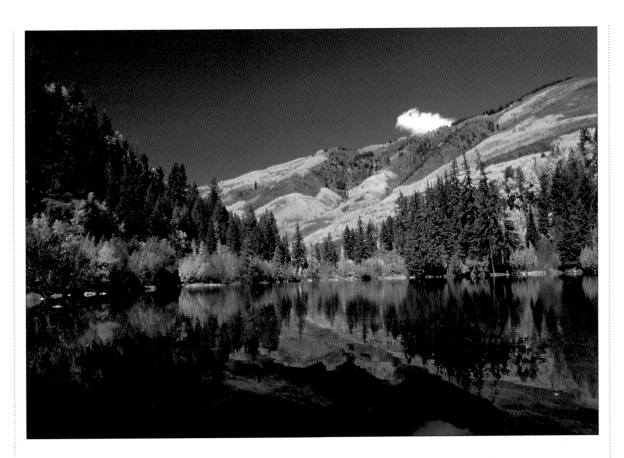

treating symptoms. Symptoms are our body's way of signalling that something is wrong and needs attention. By choosing natural methods, we choose to become more aware, connected, and conscious.

This is a time of limited financial medical resources, and restricted availability of medical care. Herbal medicine is in the perfect position to fill the gap and treat both simple and complicated medical problems. Although the theory of herbal medicine is grounded in historical facts, it is far from folklore and there is clinical and scientific research to document its efficacy. This book outlines the many ways to use botanicals in healing in a practical and useful format. Herbs can be used as a tonic, as treatment, and as a preventative. The advantages of using an inexpensive, effective, and less toxic substance are clearly beneficial.

"What is health and healing all about?", will become our major question for the 21st century. Protection of the rain forest, and fighting pollution, is vital if we are to prevent important healing plants from becoming extinct. Herbal medicine is thought to act by creating a homeostatic (metabolically balanced) healing process, rather than a suppressive one. By doing so, it promotes a balance toward health. Herbal medicine is therefore not anti-technology, but rather for self-care. We must integrate herbal therapies with conventional and complementary treatment. This holistic care gives us the knowledge and awareness to use appropriate botanical medicines. It also gives us the understanding of the relationship between ourselves, our environment, and each other. Then as we heal ourselves, we can heal the planet.

Edward J. Linkner M.D.

By protecting the natural world we live in, and taking care not to deplete the bounty it shares with us, we can begin to improve our own health and well-being.

INTRODUCTION

The magic of plants has touched most of us. We marvel at their simple start as a seed, the pattern of their unfolding leaves, and the fragrance and delicacy of their flowers. A field of wild flowers and grasses, or a forest of leafy trees, can uplift us.

WHAT IS HERBALISM?

Herbalism is the use of plants as medicines for healing. Its traditions are as old as mankind itself, and until the 18th century it was used as the most common form of medical treatment in Europe and North America. Today, in tribal cultures and among countries with Eastern traditions such as China and India, medicinal herbs are still widely used. In more conventional medicine, pharmaceutical companies and doctors rely on plants for the basis of many drugs.

EARLY HERBALISM
The first written herbal records date back well over 5,000 years to the Sumerians, who described the use and actions of plants such as laurel, caraway, and thyme. The ancient Egyptians used garlic, coriander, mint, castor oil, and opium. References in the Old Testament also speak of the use of herbal medicines.

ANCIENT CHINESE HERBALS
Chinese herbal medicine dates back to the 3rd century BC, with manuscripts found in *Ma Wang Dui* Tomb Three in Hunan province. These contained references to over 250 medicinal substances and how to use them in prescriptions. The *Yellow Emperor's Inner Classic*, compiled over 2,000 years ago, discusses the philosophical questions of health, illness, and the relationship of the human body to the cosmos. It also contains suggestions for herbs, acupuncture, diet, and exercise which are still relevant today. The traditional Chinese herbal has increased since then with the integration of substances from China's folk medicine and from other parts of Southeast Asia, India, and the Middle East.

GREEK AND ROMAN CONCEPTS
Ancient Greek and Roman medical practices are the basis for conventional medicine used in Western society today. Hippocrates, the Greek physician and "father of medicine," advocated the use of a few simple herbal drugs, along with fresh air, rest, and a healthy diet to aid the body in strengthening its own "life force" to eliminate its problems. Galen, an influential Roman physician, believed in using larger doses of the remedies, including plant, animal, and mineral substances, as the means to heal diseases. The first European treatise on the properties and uses of medicinal herbs was *De Materia Medica*, written in the 1st century AD by the Greek physician Dioscorides. It was used well into the 17th century.

THE MIDDLE AGES
The use of plants for medicines was common practice during the Middle Ages. The early Christian

church discouraged this, preferring faith healing. However, the diligent work of the monks preserved many Greek medical manuscripts, and the monasteries, with their herb gardens, became local centers for herbal treatment. Folk medicine continued the use of herbal traditions, with knowledge held by midwives and "wise women." Fear and superstition were rife, with many magical properties attached to herbal medicine. Ultimately this led to the persecution and death of many women, healers, and witches. The use of herbs was passed on through apprenticeship and word of mouth. Consequently, a great loss of herbal tradition occurred during the Inquisition, when many herbalists were put to death.

WESTERN HERBALISM

Despite the move in the 19th century toward the use of sophisticated drugs, 80 per cent of the world's population depends on medicines derived from traditional plant remedies. The recognition of the importance of ancient herbal traditions is increasing as people seek to find a greater understanding of themselves and their connection with the world around them.

THE BALANCING NATURE OF HERBS

Plants take up substances from the earth and convert them into vitamins, minerals, carbohydrates, proteins, and fats that our bodies use for nourishment and healing. By using the whole plant or herb, we take in all the vital ingredients it carries. Most herbs contain several active substances, one of which usually dominates and determines its choice as a remedy. Other healing aspects of the herb should not be overlooked because they help the body to assimilate its benefits and buffer any side-effects.

HERB COMBINATIONS

Herbs work synergistically, so combining them enhances each herb's properties, helping to bring greater healing to the body. For example, a good mixture to help induce sleep combines passiflora, valerian, and hops. All three herbs have relaxant properties, but passiflora specializes in aiding sleep, valerian relaxes muscle tension, and hops have a marked effect on relaxing the nervous system.

CHINESE HERBALISM

Chinese herbs are rarely used on their own; more commonly they are used in combination to form a Chinese prescription. The use of many herbs helps to achieve a balance within the prescription, and ensures that it enters the part of the body that needs healing. Herbs are described in terms of temperature, taste, what they do in the body, and whether they affect the *yin*, *yang*, *qi*, or blood.

YIN AND YANG

The concept of *yin* and *yang* is part of Chinese philosophy. It states that all systems of the universe consist of two conflicting yet interdependent energies from which all forms of creation came. The nature of *yang* is hot, bright, upward, and active, embodying the more masculine energy. The *yin* holds the cool, moist, inward, and nourishing qualities, which are the more feminine principles. Astragalus is a *yang* herb used to warm, strengthen and raise the *qi*, or energy. Lycium fruit is a *yin* herb whose actions go deep into the body, working to restore depleted functions and to prevent further deterioration.

QI AND BLOOD

In terms of Chinese medicine, *qi* is an energy which manifests simul-

Herbal treatments have been known and used for many centuries.

taneously on the physical, emotional, and spiritual levels, and is in a constant state of change. It is the vital force of life. Blood is seen as a denser, more material form of *qi*. *Qi* generates, moves, and holds blood, yet blood nourishes *qi*, or, as the Chinese saying goes, "Blood is the mother of *qi*." Ginseng (*ren shen*) tonifies the *qi* of the body, including that of the lungs, digestion, and heart. Chinese angelica (*dang gui*) tonifies and moves the blood (it actually strengthens the *qi* of the blood).

COMBINING WESTERN AND CHINESE HERBALISM

In this book, remedies include both Chinese and Western herbal suggestions. They can be used together safely as long as you consider any cautions and contraindications, and use safe dosages. Many Chinese remedies are given as patent remedies, and in their pill form can be used easily and safely over a period of time. Western herbal teas can be drunk at the same time to help treat any ailment. Herbal tinctures are another easy way of combining Chinese and Western herbs.

THINKING HOLISTICALLY

By recognizing that there is a link between our mind and body, and to the world around

us, we start to understand the importance of holistic health. By healing ourselves

through working closely with gifts from nature, we learn to care for the environment.

HERBS AND THE ENVIRONMENT

Our ecological awareness is much needed to avert a crisis on the planet on which we depend for life. Increasing pollution, the destruction of the rainforests, and the greenhouse effect could all have a potentially disastrous effect on us. Some herbs, which are more commonly seen as weeds, are remarkably resilient. Any gardener knows that nettles, dock, and couchgrass proliferate in most conditions. However, the more obscure healing plants are being lost as their environment is destroyed. Nature's gifts for the healing of our more serious conditions, such as cancer and AIDS, are disappearing as we wipe out traditional tribal societies, losing their knowledge, lands, and the plants they grow.

LIVING IN HARMONY WITH NATURE

We need to find a way of living in harmony with the world around us to ensure a good quality of life. Plants provide us with oxy-gen through photosynthesis, as well as food and drink, shelter, wood for coal and fuel, and medicines. From us they receive carbon dioxide, help with pollination, and bacteria to break down dead remains and return their substances into the soil, which is the place of new life. As we strengthen our life force through connection with the plants and the world around us, we become more aware of our own vitality (or lack of it) and can find healing for ourselves.

THE LIFE FORCE

The concept of the force of life is central to the philosophy of holistic healing. It is the essence that helps the body to heal itself. It is known in Chinese medicine as *qi*, and in other systems of medicine as the vital energy, or *prana*. In an holistic approach, illness occurs when there is a disturbance within this life force. Symptoms of an illness help us to identify what we need in our lives to recover and restore our own healing energy.

THE BODY IN HEALTH
For many of us it may be difficult to remember a time when we felt alive and vital. Childhood, or a long holiday, may have included moments when we felt a strong spark of life. Everyday life puts its demands on us, and we cope with them, putting aside the minor complaints of our bodies. It is when these complaints stop us from doing what we want to do that we seek help. By living in an unpolluted environment, eating a healthy diet, getting physical exercise, finding peace of mind and a positive attitude, you can do a great deal to restore good health. Herbal medicine offers much, helping us to take responsibility for our own health, and offering simple treatments. Today, in North America, increasing numbers of Holistic Physicians combine conventional and alternative therapies in the prevention and treatment of diseases.

ENVIRONMENTAL FACTORS
A pollution-free environment is hard to find these days, and is not practical for everyone. It is important to know the effect of pollution on your body. Some people are obviously more sensitive, such as asthmatics, and they need to take extra care when pollution levels are high. Herbal treatments may help to boost immunity and calm reactions to environmental factors, but a long-term environmental solution is also needed.

DIET
Food is an essential part of life, and a good diet goes a long way in preventing serious illness. A wholefood diet of preferably organic foods will help support good health. Fresh fruit and vegetables are necessary to supply essential vitamins and minerals and the roughage needed to clear wastes from the body. Avoid eating excessive amounts of foods high in refined sugars and flours, such as cakes, cookies, and candy, as well as coffee, tea, alcohol, and tobacco.

EXERCISE
Our society has become more technological; the physical exercise that was once part of everyday life has been replaced by modern conveniences. Exercise has become an optional form of recreation. This is fine, but we must make a point of exercising because it helps us to relax and release tension, build up muscle tone, and strengthen our heart and lungs. It encourages the circulation of the blood and lymph systems, so all parts of our body are warm, and our immunity is enhanced.

PEACE OF MIND
Our physical, emotional, and mental health are strongly connected. Many physical ailments, such as headaches, digestive complaints, and low immunity, are linked with stress. There are many herbal teas, baths, and oils listed throughout the book that help us to relax and let go of tensions. It may also be important to talk through difficult situations, and counseling can help. Relaxation through yoga, meditation, and *t'ai chi* can be beneficial for restoring peace of mind; so can simple pleasures like gardening, singing, and walking.

SPIRITUALITY
Spirituality is the belief in the greater good that is within all of us. Although in these times it can be difficult to carry this belief, the other option leaves us open to negativity, pessimism, and cynicism. A positive state of mind, which carries with it hope, an openness to different ways of being, and compassion for others and ourselves, helps to encourage good feelings about life.

DECIDING ON A HERBAL TREATMENT
There are many different ways of using herbs to provide a wide variety of treatments. Herbs can be taken as teas, wines, and syrups, or used externally as baths, creams, and lotions. The simplest and most common method is an herbal tea. Because of their increasing popularity, several of the more

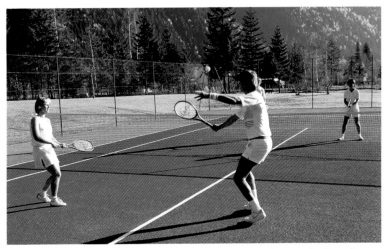

Exercise strengthens the cardiovascular system and provides a good release for everyday stress and tension.

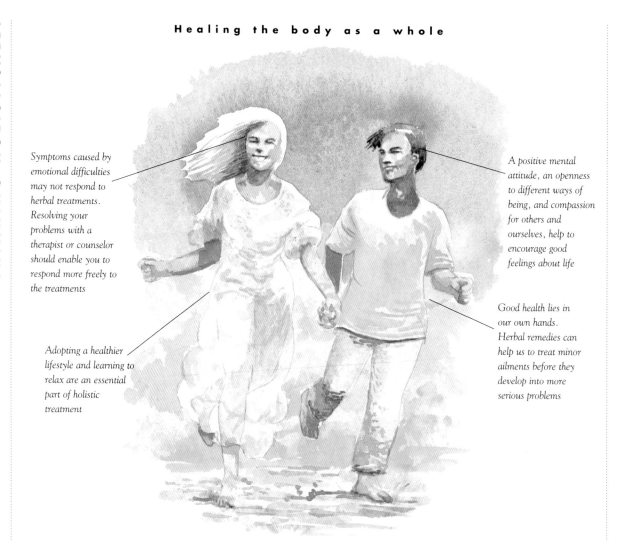

Symptoms caused by emotional difficulties may not respond to herbal treatments. Resolving your problems with a therapist or counselor should enable you to respond more freely to the treatments

A positive mental attitude, an openness to different ways of being, and compassion for others and ourselves, help to encourage good feelings about life

Adopting a healthier lifestyle and learning to relax are an essential part of holistic treatment

Good health lies in our own hands. Herbal remedies can help us to treat minor ailments before they develop into more serious problems

widely known herb teas, such as peppermint, camomile, and rose-hip, can be bought in supermarkets. If you do not enjoy their taste, try the peppermint or camomile as an essential oil in your bath!

HERBS FOR PREVENTION

Taking herbs to prevent illness and ailments is very effective and useful. Garlic and echinacea both help to boost the immune system, and are especially helpful if there is a tendency to colds or infections during the winter. If you are prone to anxiety, and know that you are facing a particularly difficult time, try drinking camomile tea to help you relax. Use lavender oil in a bath or on your pillow to help you

sleep at night so that you get a good night's rest and can cope better. Herbs can be used at the first sign of a complaint to avoid a more serious illness. Drink a hot peppermint tea with honey and a few slices of ginger root with the first sniffle of a cold, or a hot tea of boneset to ward off flu symptoms.

USING HERBS SAFELY

Herbal medicine, like any other medicine, deserves care and respect. The Herbal Directory (see pp.100–151) lists the herbs most frequently used in this book, along with any cautions or contra-indications. Take the time to look at these when you have decided on the herbs best suited for your treatment. The dosages are also

given for each herb, and must be closely followed. Standard dosages for infusions, decoctions, tinctures, wines, baths, inhalations, and Chinese patent remedies are given in the Herbal Methods section (see p.16). Remember that dosages will vary with age, so children and the elderly should take less than an adult. If a woman is breastfeeding, any herb she is taking will be excreted in her milk. It is therefore important to seek professional advice. If you are taking homeo-pathic remedies, you should consult a homeopath or herbal practitioner before beginning any herbal treatment. If you are in any doubt about using an herb, consult a professional herbalist.

HOW TO USE THIS
BOOK

This book is divided into three main sections. You may choose to read parts of it for

general interest, or consult it for treatment for different ailments. It is a reference for herbs

that may be used simply and effectively to treat a wide variety of complaints. It seeks to

give you a greater understanding of how the body works, and how to use herbal medicine.

The Body and How to Treat It   *Family name*   *The Herbal Directory*   *Common name*

Latin name

Chinese name

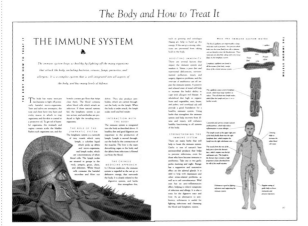

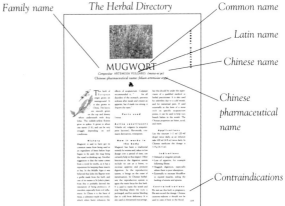

*Chinese
pharmaceutical
name*

Contraindications

HERBAL METHODS
This section describes different techniques for preparing herbs, from the making of infusions, or herbal teas, to the more complicated processes of ointments and creams. It gives useful recipes, such as an iron tonic medicinal wine that uses nettles, and an eyewash for tired eyes that contains camomile. Dosages, which will differ for the various preparations and with the age of the patient, are also given, and these must be consulted before using an herbal treatment.

THE BODY AND HOW TO TREAT IT
This section divides the body into different systems, looking at how they work and the herbal remedies that can help with their related ailments. Suggestions for preventing illness and keeping the body healthy, as well as advice regarding diet and lifestyle, are also given. Before taking any herbal treatment, check the herbs recommended in the Herbal Directory (pp. 100–151) to ensure that you are take the correct dosage and that there are no contraindications.

HERBAL DIRECTORY
This section gives specific information on the herbs recommended in this book, including a brief description of the herb, its use, how to apply it, any contraindications, and appropriate dosages. Herbs used or mentioned in the book but not included in the Directory are described briefly in the Additional Herbs list (p.152). The Glossary (p.156) explains commonly used herbal terminology. This section also includes making remedies from common items found in most kitchens, and suggestions for herbal first-aid treatments.

HERBAL METHODS

WHERE TO GET HERBS

There are several ways of obtaining herbs. The first is to pick them from the wild, following guidelines below. This will enable you to have the benefit of fresh herbs, which also can be stored and dried. Second, you can buy dried herbs from a shop, or by mail order. Third, you may decide to grow your own herbs. This will give you the advantage of being able to use fresh herbs grown right on your doorstep, as well as enjoying their foliage and scents, and reaping the medicinal benefits.

PICKING YOUR OWN HERBS

There are a few common sense rules about picking your own herbs:

- It is important to preserve the countryside and never to deplete an area of its natural resources.
- Do not uproot plants and take them home with you; it is better to select a few specimens for harvesting, and leave the rest to multiply.
- Only harvest common, plentiful plants—the weeds of the countryside—not rare or scarce plants. Be sure to check local regulations on gathering herbs.
- Always ensure that the plant you are harvesting is the plant you require—double-check, using a good field guide to wild plants.
- Better still, go on an herb walk with an experienced herbalist, who will identify plants for you.
- Above all, make sure you are not harvesting a protected species. This will ensure that nature's gifts are preserved for everyone to enjoy and benefit from.

CHOOSING HEALTHY HERBS

Check that no pesticides or herbicides have been used in the area, and that the plants are not growing close to industrial buildings or busy roads, which may throw out waste or pollution. Try and ensure that the herbs are free from animal droppings or insect damage, and are generally healthy, fresh-looking plants.

THE GROWING LIFE OF THE HERB

It is useful to familiarize yourself with the growing life of the plant you are thinking of using. Knowing the plant's habitat and growing season will add greatly to your knowledge of its medicinal value and benefits. Gather the herbs after the first dew has evaporated, but before the sun is fully on them. This will ensure they are dry, but they will not have lost any of their precious constituents.

WHICH PART OF THE PLANT TO USE

It is important to find out which part of the

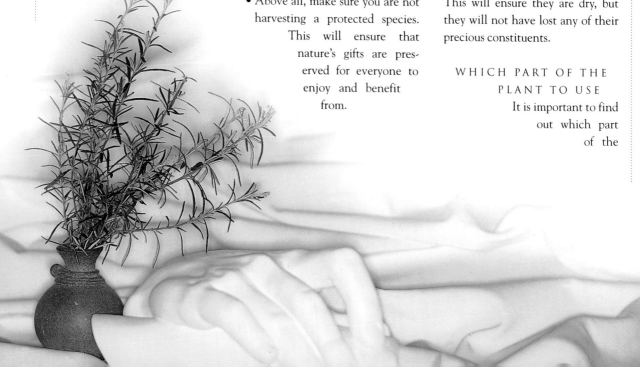

plant is best suited for your purpose. For example, while the dandelion leaf acts as a diuretic, and would be useful for those suffering from high blood pressure, the root is suitable for treating the liver, and acts as a mild laxative.

SEASONAL CHANGES

Decide which parts of the plants you intend to use, and check the time of year most suitable for harvesting them. For instance, roots are better harvested in the autumn when the aerial part of the plant has died, leaving the goodness in the roots, to be stored until spring. The leaves of a plant are best harvested in the spring. Flowers, on the other hand, are at their best later in the season. Berries should be picked when they are ripe. Bark should be purchased commercially, as cutting a tree may damage or kill it.

BUYING HERBS

You may be able to purchase dried herbs locally or from a mail order company. Either is likely to be a good source, but be sure to compare the quality by looking at, smelling, and tasting the herbs to ensure value for money. Dried herbs do not have a shelf-life of longer than about a year, so look for color: the flowers should retain some of their color and the leaves should still have some green in them; if a calendula looks pale and insipid instead of a glorious orange, it may have been sitting in storage too long. The herbs also should still have a scent. Lastly, test by taste: when infused or decocted you should be able to tell them apart; they should not taste dull or lacking in flavor.

DRYING HERBS

You can use herbs fresh, in which case you need to use them quite

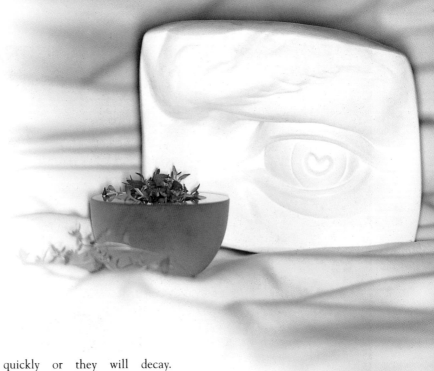

quickly or they will decay. Alternatively, you can dry the plant carefully in a warm cupboard or spread on brown paper on a rack in a warm, shady place. If drying flower heads, such as calendula, or large leaves, set them out so they do not overlap and air can circulate. Leave them to dry for one to three weeks. If mold appears it means there is too much moisture circulating and you will have to discard the batch and repeat the process. If drying a plant with smaller flowers, like lavender, or leaves, you can dry them in a paper bag, in bunches of four or five, hung upside down by their stems. Ensure that the bag covers the flower heads or leaves, then secure with an elastic band. Roots should be cleaned and cut into small pieces. Dry them in the oven on a baking tray at about 120°F (50°C) until brittle. If they remain soft, they are retaining moisture, so check them at intervals. Do be patient: too much heat too fast may destroy some of the plant's delicate constituents.

STORING HERBS

When the herbs are dry, store them in a clean, dry jar, preferably of dark glass, and keep them out of the sunlight. When buying dried herbs from a supplier, transfer them into a clean, dry jar with a close-fitting lid. Store in a dry place, out of the sunlight. Never leave herbs in plastic containers or plastic wrapping as this diminishes their shelf-life. You can store herbs in paper bags, but you need extra care to safeguard them from damp and insects. Label the container with the name of the herb and the date, or you may forget which herbs are which, and how long you have been storing them.

GROWING HERBS

If you want to buy an already growing plant, check that the specimen is from a good supplier and is healthy and free from pests. Plants that have been grown organically will be free from pesticide or herbicide residues, and will not have been grown with chemical fertilizers. This will ensure that only the most natural and healthy substances enter your body.

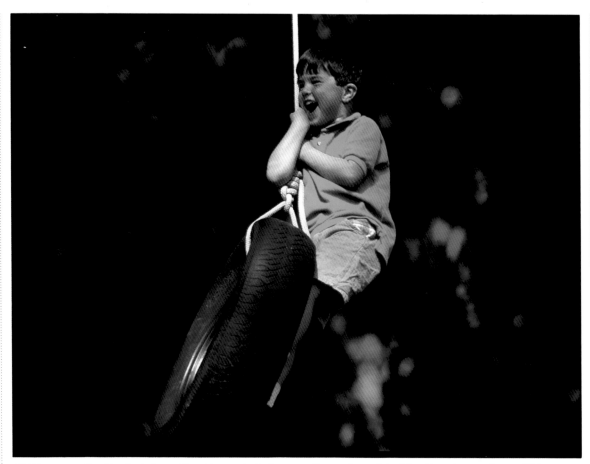

Children respond well to herbal remedies. Always check the correct dosage for each herb based on the age of your child.

DOSAGE

Dosage will depend on the method of preparation and the age of the person taking it. It is important to use just one system of measurement for dosages and recipes, so stick to metric or imperial throughout.

Infusions and decoctions are taken in cupfuls or milliliters. Each cupful is approximately 200 ml (8 fl oz) and a potful is approximately 600 ml (1¼ pints).

Tinctures are given in much smaller dosages, usually teaspoons or drops. One teaspoon is 5 ml and one milliliter is about 20 drops.

Medicinal wines are usually taken as one sherry glassful (approximately 70 ml) a day.

Syrups are taken by the teaspoonful. Between one and two teaspoons may be taken three times a day.

Guidelines for dosages

Babies to six months	Should only have herbal remedies under guidance of an experienced practitioner.
Babies to one year	One-tenth of adult dose. If the mother is breastfeeding the infant will receive the correct amount if the mother takes the normal dosage. It is important to consult a qualified practitioner.
Children one to six	One-third the normal adult dose.
Children six to twelve	One-half the normal adult dose.
Adults	Infusions 3–4 cups* a day Decoctions 2–3 cups a day Tincture 5 ml (1 tsp) 2–3 times a day
Over 70s	Infusions 2–3 cups a day Decoctions 1–2 cups a day Tincture 5 ml (1 tsp) 2–3 times a day *A cup is approximately 200 ml (8 fl oz)
Pregnancy:	Many herbs are useful in pregnancy, but it is advisable to check all remedies with a qualified practitioner before use.

INFUSIONS

Infusions are used to prepare the delicate parts of a plant, such as the leaves, flowers, and seeds, which break down easily to release their medicinal elements into the water. An infusion is also known as a tea or a tisane, a time-honored method of preparing herbs.

MAKING AN INFUSION

If making the tisane in a pot, do not use a pot used for making regular tea because the tannin will overpower the ingredients in the herbal tea. If you are making your tea in a teacup, you will need to cover it with a lid or a saucer. This is because some of the constituents of the tea include volatile oils, which evaporate in steam, and so the tea will lose much of its medicinal value if left uncovered. The tea may be drunk hot or left to cool, then placed in the refrigerator and drunk during the day. It may be kept for up to 24 hours.

Method

When using a teapot, you will need about 600 ml (1¼ pints) of boiling water, and approximately 20 g (1 oz) of dried, or 30 g (1½ oz) of fresh, herbs.

This will make enough tea to have three or four cups in a day. You may use a single herb, or a selection of two or three of equal proportions, made up to the above amount.

If using a cup, use approximately 2 g (1–2 tsp) of dried, or 3 g (2–3tsp) of fresh, herbs per cup.

Drink a cup two or three times a day, depending on what dose is appropriate (*see* p.16).

To prepare a pot of tea, first warm the vessel, then place the herbs in the pot and add freshly boiled water. Replace the lid and leave to steep for 10 minutes. Using a tea-strainer, pour the tea into a cup, adding honey as a sweetener if required. To make a single cup, place the herbs in a tea-strainer on the cup and pour over freshly boiled water until it rises up and covers the herbs. Cover and leave for 10 minutes, adding honey if desired.

COLD AND FLU TEA

one-half yarrow
one-half elderflower
pinch of peppermint
This cold and flu remedy, suitable for adults, will lower a fever, reduce nasal catarrh, and promote sweating to help cleanse and restore the system.

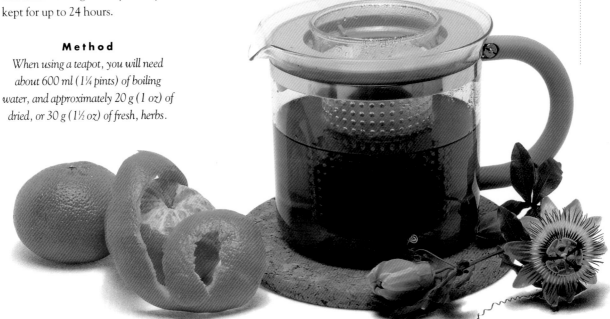

When selecting appropriate herbs for your infusion it is good to select one which adds a pleasant taste, such as lemon balm, so that your tea is refreshing as well as healthy.

DECOCTIONS

A decoction is used to prepare the more resilient parts of a plant —

the bark, roots, rhizomes, and berries — where the constituents in the

herb are more difficult to extract. Decoctions are always boiled for a

minimum of 10 minutes.

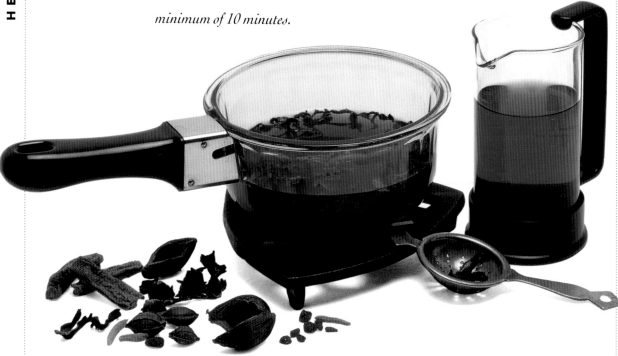

Method
20 g (1 oz) of dried, or 40 g (2 oz)
fresh, herbs to about 800 ml
(1½ pints) of water

Sections of root or bark should be chopped as finely as possible in order to allow the boiling water to extract the maximum from the plant. Place in a pan and cover with cold water, and bring to a boil. Cover the pan with a tight-fitting lid and simmer for the required period. Allow the preparation to cool before straining, pressing out as much liquid from the residue as possible in order not to waste any of the valuable properties extracted.

If you wish to combine the properties of two herbs, for example, a root and a flower or leaf, the leaf should be added at the end of the simmering period. The mixture should then be left, covered, for 10 minutes. It is possible to keep this mixture for the same period as a normal decoction because the liquid has been sterilized.

STRESS AND ANXIETY DRINK
one-third valerian root decoction
one-third skullcap infusion
one-third verbena infusion
This remedy for adults is helpful during times of stress. It will lessen anxiety, and provide a tonic for the nervous system.

Decoctions are made in larger quantities and last longer than infusions because the boiling process sterilizes the liquid.

TINCTURES

&

Tinctures can be used to prepare roots or leaves. They include alcohol and water to extract properties from the herbs which would not be available if a water preparation alone was used. It is possible to replace the alcohol with glycerol or vinegar.

STORAGE AND DOSAGE

As a tincture will last for up to two years, it is a very convenient method if you intend long-term use of the herbs. A tincture is much stronger than either an infusion or a decoction, and is taken in milli-liters (ml) or teaspoons (tsp) depending on the herb used. Use a dropper to measure amounts. In general, 20 drops = 1 ml. The average dose will vary between 1 ml (⅕ tsp) three times a day, and 5 ml (1 tsp) three times a day, but this will depend on the herb, so always check the individual herbal dosages (*see* Herbal Directory).

Method
200 g (8 oz) dried herb
250 ml (½ pint) alcohol*
750 ml (1½ pints) water
*The alcohol should be at least 30 per cent proof in order to extract constituents and to preserve them. Suitable mediums include gin and vodka. Never use industrial alcohol.

The ratio of herb to liquid is one part herb to one part liquid. The liquid is made up of 25 per cent alcohol and 75 per cent water.

Finely chop the herbs and place them in a glass vessel or jar with a tightly fitting lid. Cover the herbs with the liquid and secure the lid. The jar should be placed in a warm, dark place for 14 days. Shake the mixture every two or three days. At the end of this time, strain the mixture into a clean jar, keeping the remains of the wet herbs to one side. These can be pressed to extract every drop of the tincture by using a wine press if you have one, or by wrapping the herbs in a muslin cloth and wringing out the last few drops. Keep the tincture in a colored glass jar or bottle, and store in a dark place.

TINCTURE FOR SLEEPLESSNESS
100 g (4 oz) German camomile
250 ml (½ pint) vodka
750 ml (1½ pints) water
This tincture is excellent as an aid to restful sleep. Begin by taking 5 ml (1 tsp) approximately 20 minutes before going to bed. If this is not effective take a further 5 ml (1 tsp). You may take a maximum of 3 tsp (15 ml) in one night. The next evening you could begin with 10 ml (2 tsp) and so on until you find the most effective dose for your needs.

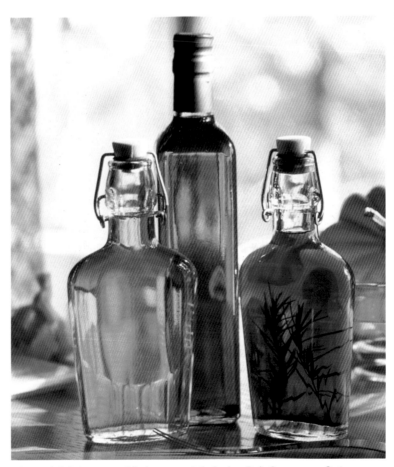

Always label tinctures with the name of the herb and the date prepared. A notebook is useful to record ailments treated and successful herbal combinations.

MEDICINAL WINES

Wines have long been used for medicinal purposes. There are two

main ways to make a medicinal wine. The first is to use a

commercially bought wine—preferably organic—and steep herbs

in it. The second is to make the wine yourself.

Method 1
100 g (4 oz) dried herbs
1 liter (2 pints) red or white wine

Place the herbs in a glass jar with a tight-fitting lid and cover with the wine. Once sealed, the jar should be left for at least two weeks to steep. The liquid should then be filtered and the liquid rebottled and stored for use as required.

Method 2
1 whole root ginger, peeled
1 kg (2¼ lb) sugar
rind and juice of 2 lemons and
2 oranges
1 banana
good pinch cayenne
pepper
200 g (8 oz) raisins
or golden raisins
yeast compound
1 large pot of tea

First squeeze the oranges and lemons, then slice the banana. Grate the ginger. Chop lemons and oranges, and add the raisins, cayenne pepper, and 450g (1 lb) of sugar. Place in a demijohn. Make a large pot of regular tea and pour over the ingredients in the demijohn. Allow the sugar to dissolve and the mixture to cool slightly, then add a general-purpose yeast compound. Loosely stopper the demijohn. Leave to ferment for at least a week, adding tea until the demijohn is about two-thirds full. Then strain the fruit and ginger and replace the liquid. Add the rest of the sugar and top-up with tea if necessary. Continue to ferment for another week, then bottle.

This wine combines the qualities of ginger and cayenne. Ginger is a warming, circulatory stimulant. It is excellent for colds as it is anti-inflammatory, antiseptic, and helps to stop coughing. Cayenne is recommended for sore throats and as a remedy for poor circulation.

CHESTY COUGH REMEDY (METHOD 1)
100 g (4 oz) dried elecampane root (or
200 g (8 oz) fresh elecampane root)
1 liter (2 pints) white wine
This tonic wine is useful for a persistent chesty cough as it both soothes inflamed tissue, and is an expectorant.

IRON TONIC RECIPE (METHOD 1)
50 g (approx. 2 oz) dried nettle
50 g (approx. 2 oz) chopped apricots
1 liter (2 pints) red wine
This wine can be used as a tonic for anemic conditions where there is lethargy and tiredness, and also for dry eczema.

Red wines are believed to have a beneficial effect on the heart while white grapes are thought to be good for the immune system, "mopping up" unwanted toxins.

GARGLES AND MOUTHWASHES

A gargle or mouthwash can be made from an infusion, a decoction, or a diluted tincture. It may be used for a variety of complaints associated with the mouth and throat. A gargle may help to soothe a sore and irritated throat associated with a cold or laryngitis.

need further treatment, for example, for a depleted immune system.

Methods

INFUSIONS/ DECOCTIONS

Make an infusion of herb tea, allow to stand for 10 minutes, then leave to cool as required. Strain, and use as a gargle or mouthwash.

TINCTURES

Dilute 5 ml (1 tsp) of the chosen tincture in 100 ml (4 fl oz) of water, and use as indicated.

MOUTH ULCER RECIPE

2 ml (½ tsp) sage tincture
2 ml (½ tsp) calendula tincture
1 ml (⅓ tsp) myrrh tincture
100 ml (4 fl oz) water
This preparation can be used either as a mouthwash when diluted, or neat as a lotion to dab directly on to the ulcers using a piece of cotton. It combines antiseptic and wound-healing properties, and is an excellent remedy for mouth ulcers. When used neat the tincture may sting slightly.

MOUTH- FRESHENING RECIPE

1 cup sage tea
A simple infusion of sage is ideal to relieve a sore throat, or simply to refresh the mouth. The volatile oils in sage help to cleanse and protect against bacteria, which can cause infection and damage teeth or gums.

A mouthwash or gargle made from an infusion, decoction, or diluted tincture can be used to keep breath fresh and to relieve tender gums or troublesome mouth ulcers.

ANTISEPTIC PROPERTIES

Choose herbs that are known for their antiseptic properties. It is safe to swallow some of the liquid as you are gargling, bearing in mind the daily recommended dosage of the herb used and any general cautions (*see* Herbal Directory). A gargle may be used four or five times a day. Where there is persistent gum trouble, seek further help from your dentist or doctor to rule out any underlying problems. If mouth ulcers continually recur, this can suggest a problem which may

EYEWASHES

An eyewash or bath can be a refreshing way to relieve tired eyes

caused by working under artificial lights and at computer screens.

An eyewash can also relieve irritation caused by

pollen or pollution.

HYGIENE

To ensure no bacteria come into contact with the eyes, all utensils, such as eyebaths, must be sterilized by boiling for 10 minutes before use. If you have only one eyebath, treat one eye, then re-sterilize the eyebath before bathing the other eye so that infection is not passed on. Better still, keep two on hand.

PREPARING AN EYEBATH

The eyebath is prepared in the same way as an infusion, but first boil the water for 10 minutes before pouring it over the herbs to be sure the water is sterilized. The liquid needs to be strained very carefully to avoid particles from the herbs being transferred to the eyes. Allow the liquid to cool before applying. If using eyebaths frequently, add a little salt to the bath to help re-balance the eye's natural fluid.

USING THE EYEBATH

Place the liquid in the eyebath and cover the eye, tipping the head back to allow the solution to gently bathe the eye. If any discomfort or irritation occurs when using an eyebath stop treatment immediately. If an infected condition persists, seek advice from a qualified practitioner.

Method 1

Make a compress by soaking a piece of cotton or lint in the eyebath infusion. Allow to cool, and place on the eyelids for 10–15 minutes.

Method 2

Prepare an infusion as described. Leave to cool until lukewarm, then fill an eyebath and bathe eyes. Twice a day should be sufficient.

TIRED EYES REMEDY (METHOD 1)

1 cup camomile tea
This is a refreshing way to ease sore or tired eyes after a hard day at work, especially if looking at a computer screen. Camomile has anti-inflammatory properties to soothe and revitalize your eyes.

CONJUNCTIVITIS REMEDY (METHOD 2)

½ cup eyebright tea
½ cup calendula tea
This remedy combines eyebright to reduce inflammation, and calendula for its antiseptic, healing qualities.

Care for your eyes by taking time out to relieve stress and tension. Use an eyebath or compress to relax and restore vitality to your eyes.

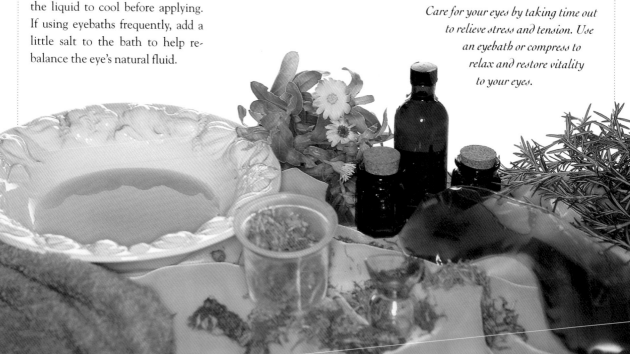

BATHS

Baths can be cleansing, relaxing, or revitalizing. When you add

herbs to your bath, you can enhance the benefits of your usual

bathtime routine. Either infusions or decoctions can be used in baths

or you may wish to try the benefits of essential oils.

If a whole-body bath is not possible, for example, in cases of illness or infirmity, a hand or foot bath can provide relief.

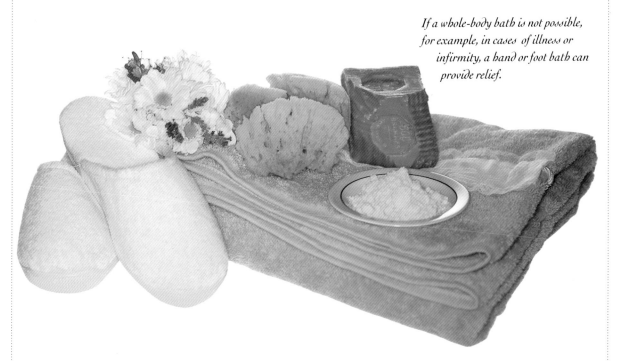

WHOLE-BODY BATH

To your normal bath water add the equivalent of one potful, or about 600 ml (1¼ pints), herbal infusion which has been strained. Mix well. Alternatively, add roughly five drops essential oils to the bath while the water is running. (Do not use essential oils in baby baths as they can ingest the oils through mouth/hand contact.) This eases aching muscles and limbs. You should not allow the bath to become too cold or the benefits will be lost. Try an infusion of lavender to relax in the evening, rosemary to invigorate in the morning, and thyme to soothe aching muscles.

HAND BATH

Using a suitable bowl or basin, immerse the whole hand up to the wrist in the cooled, strained herbal infusion. Make sure your position is comfortable: Do not sit with your hand and wrist at an awkward angle, but allow it to rest in a relaxed manner. For hot, painful arthritic joints, a cooling infusion such as peppermint is indicated, while for a cold, aching joint, a hotter infusion of ginger is warming. At all times, however, you should feel relaxed. The immersion should last between 5 and 10 minutes. Finally, make sure you dry your hands thoroughly after the bath.

FOOT BATH

This is especially good for relaxing tired, aching feet at the end of a long day. Treating your feet will enable the rest of your body to feel the benefits as well. One of the simplest remedies for a cold is to sit with your feet in a bowl of fairly hot water to which a heaped teaspoon of mustard powder has been added. Sit for 10 minutes, then dry and wrap the feet warmly.

BODY WASH

Prepare an infusion of your chosen herb, strain, and, using a clean cloth, gently bathe the selected area. Tepid water is best for this type of wash. Dry gently.

INHALATIONS

A steam inhalation can be used to relieve conditions such as colds and flu, catarrh, sinusitus, and many other problems. The steam helps to relax the airways, and benefit mucous membranes.

Method

Two potfuls (1 liter [2 pints] approximately) of liquid are needed. Prepare the infusion of herb by adding the freshly boiled water, then pour immediately into a suitable bowl placed ready for use. (It is best to take the infusion to the bowl rather than carrying a heavy, rather hot, bowl from room to room.) If using essential oils, first boil the water and pour into the bowl, then add between three to six drops of the oil to the liquid and stir. Sit comfortably and place a large towel or cloth over your head and the bowl so that none of the steam escapes. Continue this treatment for about 10 minutes or until the water cools, but do come up for air if you need to! Afterwards, sit in a warmed room for about half an hour to allow your respiratory system to adjust to the outside temperature.

CONGESTION RECIPE
2 drops thyme essential oil
2 drops eucalyptus essential oil
1 liter (2 pints) water
The properties of thyme make it an excellent decongestant for a stuffy or blocked nose or sinuses, for example, in allergic conditions. Eucalyptus oil contains ingredients which help to relax tight airways and aid breathing, as well as having antiseptic properties that are particularly good for flus and colds.

VAPORIZERS/ DIFFUSERS

If you wish to use a less-concentrated inhalation, an oil vaporizer/diffuser placed in a room is ideal. Vaporizers are easy to find, and come in many different designs and shapes. Generally, they consist of a small nightlight candle with a bowl above, into which the water and essential oil are poured. It is important to fill the bowl. A half filled bowl may crack because the light will continue to burn after the water has evaporated. Use between 1 and 6 drops of essential oil. If a vaporizer is not available, a bowl filled with boiling water to which the essential oil is added will allow the vapour to diffuse throughout the room. Or a drop or two of oil on a piece of cotton or clean cloth placed above (not on) a radiator will have much the same effect.

TENSION RECIPE
3–5 drops lavender essential oil
bowl of hot water/diffuser
Lavender has a calming, sedative effect. If tension prevents you from winding down after a hard day, add this to a bowl of water or a diffuser, and allow your cares to drift away.

HERBAL HEALING
The addition of an herbal remedy to a steam inhalation helps to ease congestion, clear mucus, and relieve respiratory stress. Younger children with colds may benefit from being taken into a steamy bathroom to ease breathing and other symptoms.

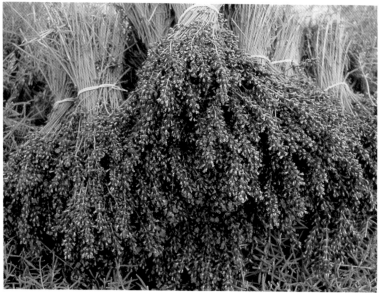

Lavender has a calming, sedative effect. Use it as an essential oil in a steam inhalation to relieve a headache caused by stress and to aid restful sleep.

INFUSED OILS

Infused oils are altogether different from essential oils and can be made easily and cheaply at home. They can be used for massage or as a base oil to which essential oils can be added.

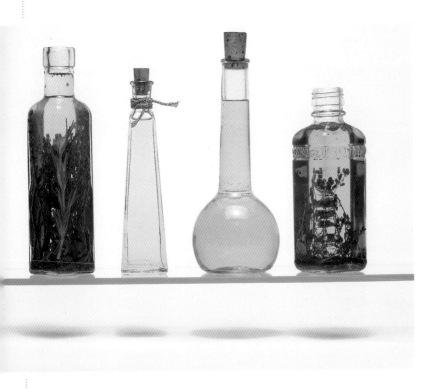

Hot and cold oil infusions can be used for massage and also as a base when making creams and ointments.

WHICH OILS TO USE
The best oils for infusions are vegetable, either sunflower or soya, for example. Use olive oils only for cold infusions. Oils will last for about a year.

CAUTION
Handle hot oils carefully. *Never* use oils internally or allow them to come into contact with delicate membranes, such as the eyes.

COLD AND HOT OILS
There are two ways of making an infused oil: a cold preparation where the oils are heated by the sun, and a hot preparation where the oils are heated gently on the stove.

Method
COLD OILS
This method is very easy but slow. First, obtain a clean, dry jar with a tight-fitting lid and pack it full with your chosen herb. Gently pour the oil into the jar, covering the herbs fully. Put the lid on and place it on a warm, sunny windowsill for about two weeks, shaking and turning the jar daily. At the end of this time you will need to strain the oil carefully, using a muslin bag or cloth stretched over a bowl. Make sure all the plant material is removed, and squeeze out every last drop of oil to get the maximum benefit. Store your oils in dark bottles away from sunlight. Do not forget to label and date your preparation.

HOT OILS
*100 g (4 oz) dried herb
or 200 g (8 oz) fresh herb
400 ml (16 fl oz) vegetable oil*

This process is somewhat more complicated but gives a good-quality oil. The method uses a double boiler—a pan filled with water, brought to a boil and gently simmering, over which a larger pan or glass bowl is placed. The vegetable oil and herb are put into this, so the oil never comes into direct contact with the heat. The pan or bowl containing the oil and herb should be covered with a tight-fitting lid. The mixture is then left for a minimum of two hours, and allowed to cool before filtering the oil into a clean bowl, using a cloth or straining bag. The used herb should be discarded and the process repeated, using fresh herbs, thus giving a double strength to your oil. Again, at the end, the oil should be filtered and the used herb thrown away. Bottle your oil in dark glass jars, and store out of the sunlight.

NERVE TONIC OIL
*St John's wort flowers
vegetable oil
The flowers of St. John's wort are yellow, but as the plant oils are diffused into the vegetable oil, the color will turn deep red. This oil is excellent for gently massaging into areas where there is nerve strain or pain, for example, in cases of repetitive strain injury or neuralgia.*

OINTMENTS

Ointments are oil-based preparations which, in addition to aiding the healing process, form a protective layer on the skin. This makes them ideally suited for use where areas of skin are exposed to the elements, for example, chapped lips or dry eczema.

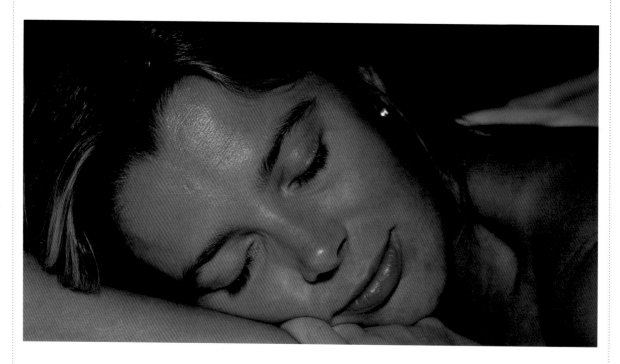

PATCH TEST FOR SENSITIVE SKIN

Homemade herbal creams and ointments are ideal for those with sensitive or allergic skin because you can choose your own ingredients and minimize the use of additives or preservatives which can cause irritation. However, before using any remedy on the skin first try a patch test. Apply a little of the ointment or cream on to an area of skin and leave it for 24 hours. If any reaction occurs, discontinue use. Seek medical advice if the irritation persists.

Method
200 ml (8 fl oz) infused oil
25 g (1 oz) beeswax
2–5 drops essential oil

Fill a pan with water, bring to a boil and then reduce to a simmer. Place another pan or glass bowl over the boiling water and pour in the oil. Grate the beeswax into small pieces and add gradually, stirring until the wax is melted. Add any essential oils you wish to use. Remove the bowl from the heat, and, while still warm, carefully pour into a clean glass jar and allow to set. Seal the jar, then label and date it.

Homemade ointments and creams provide a gentle alternative to commercially made products. They can bring relief to skin that has been affected by sun, age, food, and soap.

OINTMENT FOR CUTS AND SCRAPES
200 ml (8 fl oz) infused calendula oil
25 g (1 oz) beeswax
2 drops lavender essential oil
This ointment combines the anti-bacterial healing properties of calendula with the astringent and anti-inflammatory qualities of lavender.

CREAMS

✿

Skin creams are preparations which combine oil and a water-based

medium to create a mixture which nourishes and enriches the skin.

Creams that are firm act as a barrier against the elements, while

those of liquid consistency can be used to cleanse and moisturize.

PREPARING A CREAM

Creams are slightly more difficult to prepare than ointments since the oil and water base must be carefully blended or the two ingredients will separate out. The water base portion of the recipe could be either an infusion or a decoction of the chosen herbs. An agent is required to facilitate the blending process, usually emulsifying wax.

HOW MUCH TO MAKE

Because a cream includes water, its shelf-life will be less than an ointment, therefore it is better to prepare only a small quantity. To help preserve and enhance the quality of the cream it is possible to add an essential oil. A cream should always be stored in a cool place or in the refrigerator.

Method

7 parts infusion/decoction
2 parts oil
1 part emulsifying wax

This ratio is always the same whatever the amounts you are using. If you are using teaspoons, the recipe will use seven teaspoons of infusion, two teaspoons of oil, and one teaspoon of emulsifying wax. Mix in three drops of essential oil to each 30 g (1½ oz) jar made. Fill a pan with water, bring to a boil, and simmer. Place a second pan or bowl over the first and pour in the oil and infusion. Gradually add in the emulsifying wax, stirring until it is dissolved. Remove the bowl from the heat, and place in a bowl filled with cold water. It is important to keep stirring the mixture as it cools or the ingredients will separate out. As it cools, the cream will take on a thicker consistency. Add the essential oil and mix well. Spoon the mixture into glass jars, replace the lids, label, and date. Store in the refrigerator or a cool place.

SOOTHING CREAM

7 teaspoons chickweed infusion
2 teaspoons oil
1 teaspoon emulsifying wax
3 drops camomile essential oil
Chickweed is extremely cooling and is noted for its effective relief of itching. Camomile essential oil combines anti-allergenic and anti-inflammatory properties with the preservation and enhancement of the fragrance of the cream.

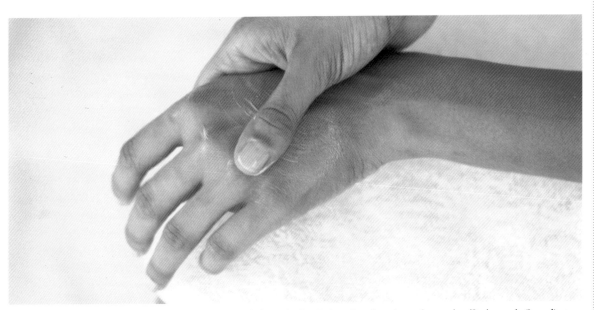

Creams are particularly good for soothing an area of skin which is irritated or dry. A patch test should always be done first.

SYRUPS

Syrups are soothing mixtures which are popular with adults and children alike. You can turn an infusion, a decoction, or a tincture into a syrup by combining the liquid-based remedy with sugar or honey. This will also improve the taste of less pleasant herbs.

Method
INFUSION-BASED
SYRUP
200 ml (8 fl oz) infusion
200 g (8 oz) sugar/honey

For this type of syrup, you will need equal amounts of infusion and sugar. Prepare your infusion in the usual manner, but leave it to steep for 15 rather than 10 minutes.

Strain the tea as usual, taking care to press out as much of the liquid as possible. The liquid should then be heated gently in a pan and the sugar or honey added. Stir constantly to dissolve all the sugar, taking care not to boil the mixture. Allow the syrup to cool, then pour into bottles, seal, and label. Store in a cool, dark place. (Take care when sealing that the lid is left slightly loose as tightly stoppered bottles have been known to explode.)

Method
DECOCTION-BASED
SYRUP

This method is exactly the same as for infusion-based syrups except that the decoction should be simmered for 30 minutes.

Method
TINCTURE-BASED
SYRUP
100 ml (4 fl oz) water
200 g (8 oz) sugar
100 ml (4 fl oz) tincture

First prepare the syrup, and then add the tincture. Boil the water, and then add it to the sugar or honey, which are in another pan. Stir until all the sugar is dissolved, then remove from the heat. Allow to cool, then stir in the tincture. Bottle, seal, and label as before. The quantities used are always the same ratio, that is, one part tincture to three parts syrup.

RECIPE FOR COUGH SYRUP (INFUSION)
200 ml (8 fl oz) infusion of thyme
200 g (8 oz) unrefined sugar
This remedy uses the antiseptic and expectorant qualities of thyme to relieve coughs and sore throats, and is especially good for children.

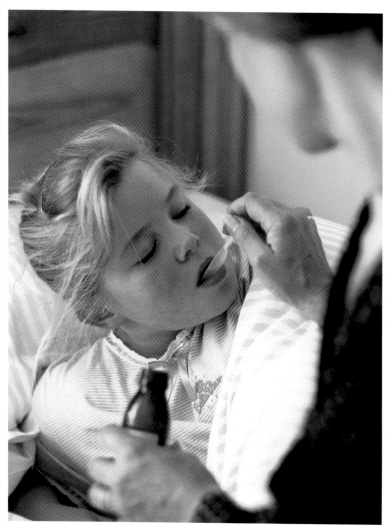

Syrups are sweet and easily swallowed so they are useful in the treatment of coughs and sore throats, particularly when treating children.

VINEGARS

Vinegars can be used in a similar way to tinctures, and can provide an alternative for those who do not find either the alcoholic or glycerine preparations suitable. Vinegar contains acetic acid, which helps to preserve and extract the essential ingredients of herbs.

PREPARATION

Use a jar or bottle with a wide mouth. Choose your herb, making sure it is as dry as possible. Place the herb in the jar and top up with the vinegar. Store for a minimum of two weeks (some sources recommend one or two months) in a dark place, shaking every day. Then strain off the liquid and bottle. The vinegar should be left for a further two weeks before using.

DOSAGE

Herb vinegars can be taken internally in the same way as tinctures, that is, by the teaspoonful, or added to salads, soups, or as an ingredient in pickles. Externally they can be added to bathwater, and used as a lotion, or even a hair rinse. The recipes given below show how versatile vinegars can be.

ITCHY-SKIN LOTION
elderflower blossoms
apple cider vinegar
The flowers of the elder tree are noted for their anti-inflammatory action. Especially valued for internal use in allergic conditions, the flowers can also be used in a vinegar-base as an external wash to calm and soothe itching skin, especially in cases of allergic reactions.

As a first-aid measure it is useful to have some on hand to alleviate the painful burning of an insect sting.

DRY-SCALP RINSE
nettle tops
white wine vinegar
The astringent properties of nettle and the softening effects of vinegar combine to help bring a shine to dull hair and encourage circulation to a dry scalp. Add a little of the vinegar to your final rinsing water.

SALAD DRESSING
2 cloves garlic, peeled and chopped
200 ml (8 fl oz) white wine vinegar
Garlic is famed for its healing properties, but its pungent odor can be problematic. Including it in a vinegar dressing and adding it to salads often proves more palatable. Medicinal benefits include an antibiotic effect and an anti-cholesterol action. It is also a good remedy for chest and other respiratory infections.

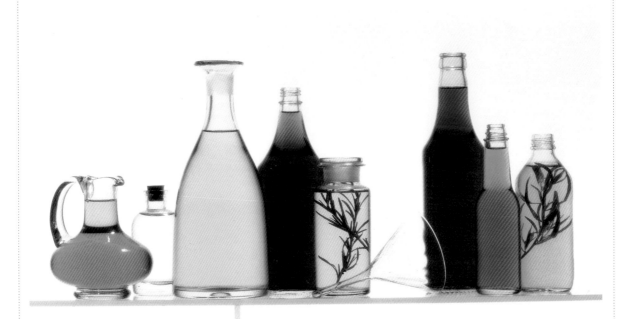

In addition to their medicinal function, vinegars are an interesting way to complement foods. Apple cider or wine vinegars, preferably organic, are most versatile.

POULTICES AND COMPRESSES

Traditionally, poultices are used to draw out toxins from the body, promote circulation, and aid healing. Poultices and compresses are applied in the same way, but are prepared differently and perform different functions.

RECIPE FOR
DRAWING PASTE
Equal parts of:
marshmallow root powder
slippery elm powder
water
This recipe combines the drawing qualities of marshmallow with the demulcent, soothing properties of slippery elm. Use it for drawing out splinters, insect stings, and boils. It can also be used to counter irritation from insect bites.

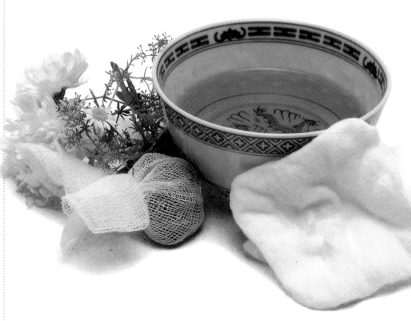

Use a cool poultice or compress for hot, inflamed conditions and a warm application to relieve strain and aching in cold, painful areas.

COMPRESSES

Compresses are also applied directly to the skin, but in this case it is the liquid from the mixture rather than the herb which is used. Again, a compress can utilize either an infusion, a decoction, or a tincture. If using a tincture, it should be diluted with a little water. For this method you will need a clean cloth for soaking in the liquid. Once the liquid portion is prepared, the cloth should be soaked thoroughly and then wrung out. As for poultices, first apply a little oil to the area to prevent sticking, and then apply the cloth to the skin. To retain moisture, cover with plastic wrap or a plastic bag, and secure with a bandage. Replace as needed.

COOLING COMPRESS
200 ml (8 fl oz) lavender infusion
A lavender compress can be placed on the forehead or the back of the neck to relieve tension and headaches.

POULTICES

A poultice is an herb applied to a particular area. You can use herbs in fresh, dried, or powdered form.

FRESH HERB POULTICE

First, apply a little sunflower or vegetable oil to the skin to prevent sticking. Crush the plant and then place it directly on to the affected area. Hold the poultice in place with a dressing or bandage.

DRIED HERB POULTICE

Dried herbs must first be decocted by placing them in a pan with water and simmering them for approximately five minutes. Allow the mixture to cool. Squeeze out the liquid and keep the remaining material. As this poultice is more difficult to apply directly, first place the herbs on to the dressing, and spread evenly.

POWDERED HERB POULTICE

First mix the powders with a cold liquid, either water or a tincture. Stir until a fine paste is created, then spread on to the bandage as described.

PESSARIES AND SUPPOSITORIES

Pessaries and suppositories can help relieve localized conditions, such as vaginal candida, thrush, and hemorrhoids. They can also be used to give an herbal remedy that may be broken down by digestion before it reaches the target area.

Method 1
10 g (½ oz) beeswax
40 g (2 oz) grated cocoa butter
100 ml (4 fl oz) oil
7 drops essential oil

Prepare a pessary mold (available from specialist suppliers) by brushing thinly with soft soap to prevent sticking (if the mold has been placed in the freezer beforehand, the mixture will set more quickly). Using a double boiler, melt the beeswax in the oil, then add the cocoa butter and stir until dissolved. Remove from the heat, add essential oil, and pour into a mold. Place in the freezer for 5 to 10 minutes, then complete the setting process by putting it into the refrigerator. When set, cut into 2.5-cm (1-in) long pellets.

Method 2
10 parts gelatin
15 parts glycerine
40 parts water-base

The ratio of this formula is always the same, that is, 10 teaspoons, 15 teaspoons, and 40 teaspoons, and so on. Soak the gelatin in the water, then dissolve on a very low heat. Add the glycerine and place in a double boiler. Allow the water to slowly evaporate until the required consistency is reached. Pour into a mold and follow the instructions given above.

HEMORRHOID SUPPOSITORIES
10 parts gelatin
15 parts glycerine
40 parts witch hazel infusion
The astringent qualities of witch hazel will help to shrink and relieve painful hemorrhoids.

Pessaries and suppositories allow herbs to be absorbed into the blood directly and utilized by the body. Keep them refrigerated as they will melt at body temperature.

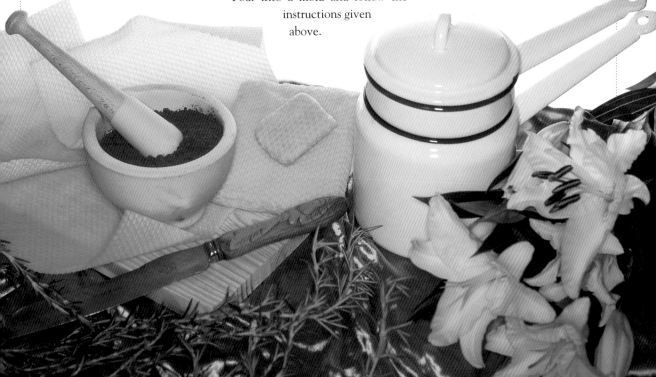

CHINESE HERBAL DECOCTIONS

Decoction (tang) literally means "soup." It is one of the most common ways of taking traditional Chinese herbal medicine. With a decoction, it is possible to create a prescription made of eight to ten herbs that is carefully balanced in its properties, and directed to a specific area of the body.

Chinese herbal decoctions generally use a greater number of herbs than Western herbal decoctions. Because the preparation of a decoction takes some time, and the cooking smell fills the house, many people prefer to use herbal tablets. However, if you wish to make your own decoctions, the guidelines below will help.

QUANTITIES

Use approximately 800 ml (1½ pints) water with 40 g (2 oz) of Chinese herbs. This will allow several herbs to be used in one decoction. The common dosage is 3–10 g (⅛–½ oz) per herb daily, but do take note of the dosages recommended for individual herbs in the Herbal Directory. Children, the elderly, pregnant women, and those with weak digestive systems must take the smaller dosage. If a Chinese herbalist includes many herbs in a prescription, a daily dosage of 80–120 g (3–4½ oz) may be given.

PREPARATION

There are a variety of ways of preparing a decoction, depending on the herbs used and the practitioner prescribing them. Always use a non-aluminum pot. Soak the herbs for two hours in enough water to cover them completely. Tonic herbs, such as astragalus (*huang qi*), Chinese angelica (*dang gui*), and licorice (*gan cao*), which are used to strengthen the system, should be simmered gently in a covered pot for one hour. Herbs for more acute conditions, such as chrysanthemum (*ju hua*), burdock (*nui bang zi*), dandelion (*pu gong ying*), and honeysuckle (*jin yin hua*), should be simmered for 20–30 minutes. Strain the herbs from the liquid and drink warm in equal doses, morning and evening.

Several Chinese herbs mentioned in this book need to be prepared differently. The volatile oils, which give these herbs their fragrance, are part of their healing qualities. Because they are easily destroyed by over-cooking, peppermint (*bo he*) and perilla leaf (*zi su ye*) should be added in the last five minutes of preparation.

GINSENG

Ginseng is another Chinese herb that is often prepared separately because of its expense. A piece of good ginseng root is worth a great deal of money, and is valued highly in China for its life-enhancing properties. Put 1–9 g (¹⁄₁₆–½ oz) ginseng in a small amount of water placed over a double boiler. Simmer for an hour, then strain off the liquid. Add this to liquid from other herbal decoctions, or drink it on its own. The ginseng root can be cooked in this way several times to get all the goodness out and to use it efficiently.

CHINESE PATENT FORMULAS

Chinese patent formulas are classical herbal prescriptions that can be taken in pill or tincture form. For this reason, they are easier to take than decoctions and have increased in popularity. These traditional formulas can be an effective treatment for a wide range of ailments.

Traditional Chinese patent formulas are still imported from China by most suppliers of Chinese herbs. Many Western manufacturers have adapted the traditional formulas to treat modern Western conditions. The Western adaptations often list the traditional formula on which the prescription is based, which is a handy reference to some of the more commonly available prescriptions.

THE CHINESE COURT

The classical Chinese herbal formulas, which have been used for many centuries, were often based on members of the Chinese court. These formulas consist of many herbs which work in balance and harmony. The Four Gentlemen Decoction (*Si Jun Zi Tang*), was derived from the Confucian term meaning an exemplary person, and the number four, whose nature is harmonious. The chief herb, also known as the emperor, or *jun* herb, is ginseng, which strengthens the *qi*, or energy, of the body.

The minister, or *chen* herb, white atractylodis rhizome (*bai zhu*), acts as the advisor, and works synergistically. The assistant, or *zuo* herb, is poria (*fu ling*), which works to balance the cloying nature of the tonic herbs to make them more digestible. The envoy or *shi* herb, honey-fried licorice (*zhi gan cao*), delivers the whole prescription to the digestive system and the 12 main channels of the body.

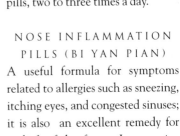

WOMEN'S PRECIOUS PILLS (BA ZHEN WAN)

This is an excellent women's tonic which combines the two classical formulas: the Four Gentlemen, which strengthens the *qi*, or energy, and the Four Substances, which nourishes the blood. It is useful in conditions of tiredness, dizziness, irregular menstruation, scanty periods, poor circulation, and in the recovery from childbirth or long-term illness. It contains the herbs listed in the Four Gentlemen Decoction and Chinese angelica (*dang gui*), which is one of the herbs in the Four Substances which strengthens the blood and improves circulation. Take five pills, two to three times a day.

NOSE INFLAMMATION PILLS (BI YAN PIAN)

A useful formula for symptoms related to allergies such as sneezing, itching eyes, and congested sinuses; it is also an excellent remedy for relief of hayfever. It contains chrysanthemum flower

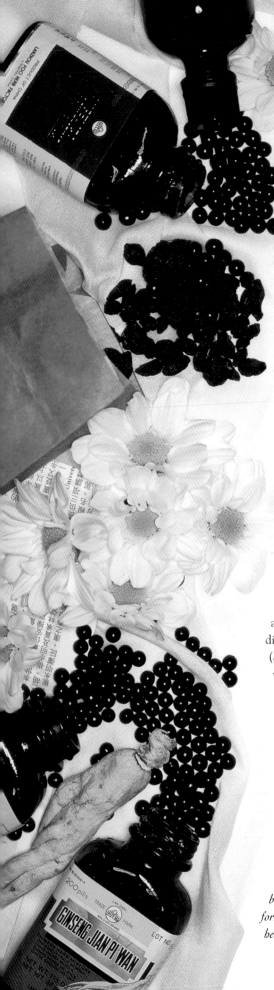

(*ju hua*) and forsythia (*lian qiao*), which help to clear the first signs of colds. Take four tablets, three times a day, one-half hour after eating.

CENTRAL QI PILLS (BU ZHONG YI QI WAN)

A useful formula helping to strengthen and invigorate the digestion. It relieves symptoms of bloating, pain, wind, and alternating constipation and diarrhea. Also helps to raise the *yang*, or lift prolapses of the uterus and rectum, hemorrhoids, and varicose veins. It contains the Chinese herbs codonopsis root (*dang shen*)—which is a less-expensive substitute for ginseng—astragalus (*huang qi*), angelica (*dang gui*), and licorice (*gan cao*), all of which help support the immune system. These herbs also help to strengthen the digestion, along with citrus peel (*chen pi*), and ginger (*sheng jiang*), which aid movement of food through the system. Take five pills, two to three times a day.

Chinese herbal patent remedies, based on traditional Chinese formulas, are a simple way of taking herbal treatments.

DECOCTION FOR FRIGID EXTREMITIES (DANG GUI SI NI TANG)

Used to warm the extremities and nourish the blood, this formula is often taken in tincture form because alcohol is warming and easily absorbed into the bloodstream. It is useful in conditions of poor circulation, rheumatoid arthritis with cold symptoms, Raynaud's disease, and frostbite. It contains Chinese angelica (*dang gui*), which strengthens the blood and improves the circulation, and cinnamon (*gui zhi*), which is warming. It should be used with caution in the spring and summer, in warm climates, or with symptoms of heat, such as fever and sweating. Take one teaspoon in warm water, three times a day.

ANGELICA AND LORANTHUS PILL (DU HUO JI SHENG WAN)

A formula used to strengthen the back and lower extremities and ease stiffness. It is helpful with low-back pain, sciatica, and arthritis, especially when the condition is helped by heat and warmth, or due to deficiency. It contains Chinese angelica (*dang gui*), which encourages circulation, and the warming herbs of ginger (*sheng jiang*), and the inner bark of the cinnamon tree—(*rou gui*). Take five pills, two to three times a day.

EAR-RINGING LEFT LOVING PILLS (ER LONG ZUO CI WAN)

A variation of *Liu Wei Di Huang Wan* (*see below*), these pills help to ease symptoms of tinnitus, headache, high blood pressure, insomnia, thirst, and eye pressure and irritation. Take five pills, three times a day; they can be taken over a period of time.

SIX-FLAVOR REHMANNIA PILL (LIU WEI DI HUANG WAN)

A classic Chinese herbal prescription, which forms the basis for other prescriptions. It is nourishing for the *yin* aspect, strengthening the liver, kidney, and spleen. It helps to ease symptoms of weakness or pain in the lower back, burning in palms or soles of the feet, mild night sweats, dizziness, tinnitus, and a mild, constant sore throat. It can help high blood pressure and diabetes, but professional advice should first be sought. Take five pills, three times a day. These may be taken over a period of time, but may aggravate catarrhal conditions.

BRIGHT EYES REHMANNIA PILLS (MING MU DI HUANG WAN)

Another variation of *Liu Wei Di Huang Wan* (*see* above) which helps to benefit many eye complaints especially in the elderly. This formula contains Chinese angelica (*dang gui*), which helps to nourish the blood and improve circulation. The herbs chrysanthemum flower (*ju hua*) and lycium fruit (*gou qi zi*) are particularly beneficial for the eyes. Take five pills, three times a day.

LYCIUM, CHRYSANTHEMUM, REHMANNIA PILLS (QI JU DI HUANG WAN)

A variation of *Liu Wei Di Huang Wan* (*see* above) which helps to treat blurry vision, poor night vision, dry and painful eyes, and pressure behind the eyes. It differs from *Ming Mu Di Huang Wan* (*see* above) in that it also treats headache, dizziness, irritability, restlessness, and insomnia. It can be helpful with menopausal symptoms. As stated in its English name, this formula contains lycium fruit (*gou qi zi*) and chrysanthemum flower (*ju hua*), which help to nourish the eyes. Take five pills, three times a day.

CLEAN AIR TEA (QING QI HUA TAN WAN)

A useful prescription for the treatment of asthma, chronic bronchitis, or sinus infection when there is a thick, sticky phlegm that is difficult to clear. Take five pills, three times a day.

MORUS, CHRYSANTHEMUM MEDICINE PILL (SANG JU YIN PIAN)

A useful pill to clear the first signs of a cough, especially a dry one, accompanied by a dry, sore throat, sneezing, runny nose, and watery eyes. It contains forsythia fruit (*lian qiao*), chrysanthemum flower (*ju hua*), and peppermint (*bo he*), all of which help to eliminate symptoms of colds and flu. Take three tablets, two to three times a day.

CODONOPSIS, PORIA, ATRACTYLODES FORMULA (SHEN LING BAI ZHU PIAN)

A useful formula for strengthening weak digestion. It helps to clear symptoms of bloating, indigestion, and loose stools. It is a good tonic for children with poor appetite and slow growth. Take five pills, three times a day. Children can take three pills, two to three times a day.

ZIZYPHUS SEED SOUP TABLET (SUAN ZAO REN TANG PIAN)

A prescription to calm the *shen* or "spirit of the heart," helping with problems of insomnia, restlessness, heart palpitations, and mental agitation. Take two tablets, three times a day.

HEAVENLY KING BENEFIT HEART PILL (TIAN WANG BU XIN WAN)

Useful to calm the *shen* in cases where there is a deficiency or chronic tiredness. It is helpful with insomnia, anxiety, palpitations, and vivid dreaming. It is also used in treating hyperactive thyroid. Take five pills, three times a day.

FREE AND EASY WANDERER (XIAO YAO WAN)

A basic formula used to nourish the blood, move the *qi*, or energy, and strengthen the digestion. It is helpful with a range of symptoms, such as bloating and fullness in the abdomen, menstrual disorders, and tension headaches. This contains Chinese angelica (*dang gui*), which is useful for many menstrual problems. Take five pills, three times a day.

LONICERA, FORSYTHIA DISPEL HEAT TABLETS (YIN QIAO JIE DU PIAN)

An excellent remedy to clear colds when taken with the first symptoms such as a sore throat, fever with chills, stiff muscles, and sneezing. This formula contains the following herbs used to dispel early symptoms of colds: peppermint (*bo he*), forsythia fruit (*lian qiao*), honeysuckle (*jin yin hua*), and burdock seed (*nui bang zi*). Take five pills, every three hours for the first nine hours, then every five hours as needed. Discontinue after three days.

THE BODY & HOW TO TREAT IT

This section describes the different systems of the body and their related ailments. Herbal treatments and methods of application are suggested so that common complaints can be treated gently but effectively.

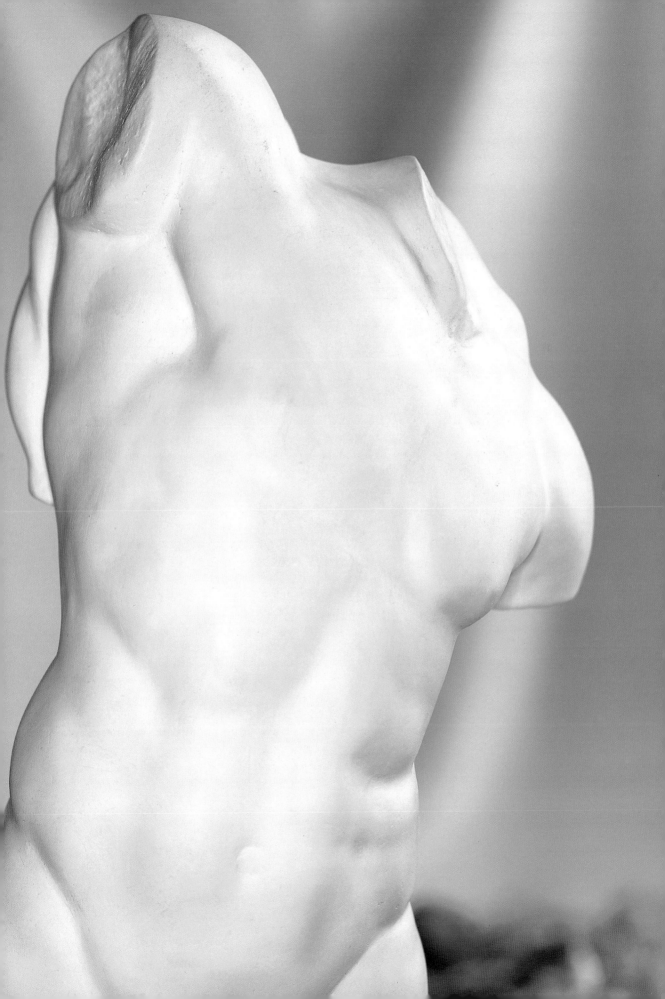

HEALING HERBS

The ability to heal ourselves, to restore and revitalize our life force, or qi, lies within us.

Plants offer simple remedies to help enhance our own healing process. Understanding

how our body works helps us to appreciate its efficiency and ability to repair itself. We

need to work with our body, not against it. Herbal medicine will help support us so we

can bring about a deeper, permanent change within ourselves.

HOW TO USE THIS SECTION

This section contains the different systems in the body and their related ailments. Within each system there will be a brief description of how it works, its interaction to the rest of the body, and how it is viewed in terms of Chinese medicine. Suggestions for preventing illnesses and complaints will also be given, including changes in diet, lifestyle, and outlook on life. Understanding the whole picture of your particular ailment will help the herbal healing process.

CHOOSING THE RIGHT HERBS FOR THE RIGHT TREATMENT

With most ailments, several suggestions for herbal treatment will be given. These will include combinations of herbs, Chinese remedies, and external herbal treatments. Before using any herbs, please check the Herbal Directory to find out more about the herb, and take care to note any cautions, contraindications, and dosages. Then read the Herbal Methods section to find out the most beneficial way of preparing the herb. If the specific dosages have not been given in the Herbal Directory, use the recommended dosages listed here. Be sure to take into account any changes in dosage for both the elderly and children.

CAUTIONS AND CONTRAINDICATIONS

Herbs are safe to use if taken in the right amount, with cautions and contraindications observed. There is much debate about herbal safety, and we have listed precautions we have found while researching this book. Pregnancy is one condition where care needs to be taken when using herbs. Digestive problems, skin complaints, and blood pressure may be aggravated with the use of certain herbs, so please check the Herbal Directory beforehand. Care must also be taken with essential oils; they should not be taken internally or used with babies. Please read the Herbal Directory carefully, and seek advice from a professional herbalist if you have any doubts about the use of an herb.

COMBINING HERBS AND DRUGS

If you are taking medication for a serious medical problem, it is best to seek advice from a professional medical herbalist and your doctor. Herbs can be used with most medications, but it is important to select the most appropriate ones. **DO NOT STOP TAKING ANY MEDICATION** without the advice of your doctor and herbalist. Be aware that taking herbs may change your need for medication, and this must be monitored regularly. For example, hawthorn berries must not be taken with certain cardiovascular medication as they will alter this, which can affect the heart.

WHEN HERBS ARE INEFFECTIVE

Herbal treatment will vary with different types of conditions. Acute infections, such as colds and flu, will need a treatment that has an immediate effect, while more chronic conditions like arthritis will need long-term treatment. Generally, you will know in a matter of days whether an acute infection is clearing, as the symptoms will become better quickly. If one herb does not work, try some of the other herbs mentioned. If no herbal treatments seem to be effective, it is probably time to call a doctor, as symptoms of acute infections such

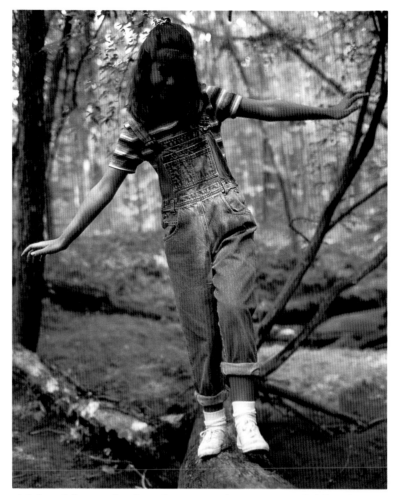

A balanced diet, regular physical exercise, and a positive attitude help to keep us healthy. Herbal medicine supports our natural flow of energy helping to gently heal us.

as fever, vomiting, or diarrhea can be debilitating and dangerous if left for more than a few days. With chronic conditions it is sometimes hard to know if the herbs are helping as the symptoms may vary from day to day. Herbal treatment may need to be over a period of several weeks, and diet and lifestyle may also require changes. If the condition generally has not improved after several weeks, you may need to go to a professional herbalist to find the right herbs.

HOME CARE AND PROFESSIONAL HERBALISM

Most of the herbal suggestions in this book are safe to use as a way of looking after ourselves, families, and friends. Herbal baths, vaporizers, and simple herbal teas can be taken as part of a daily routine that helps maintain good health and feelings of well-being. There may be times when you need professional advice from an herbalist as the condition is too serious to be undertaken without experience and training. Make sure that you go to a herbalist who is registered with a recognized professional body or institute. The herbalist will take a case history and prescribe appropriate herbs; they will also be supportive in helping you make any other changes needed.

RESPIRATION

We can only survive several minutes without breathing. The air we breathe

brings us the essential element which is vital for life: oxygen. Our

respiratory system needs to be in good working order to take in revitalizing

oxygen, and filter out the toxins that are now so much part of our environment.

Our first contact with air is through the nose and mouth. Our nose alerts us to the smell of the air – is it fresh and fragrant, or full of toxic fumes? Sometimes we can even taste the poisonous gases in the air, and our reaction may be to hold our breath for several seconds. Infectious bacteria from someone who is ill also pass through the air. Our nose, mouth, and throat are our first line of defense. They contain cilia, or tiny hairs, that cleanse the nose and throat by pulling mucus and saliva into the stomach, where it is sterilized. Saliva and mucus protect the delicate lining of the mouth and nose by trapping invasive particles. Under healthy conditions these mechanisms work very well to keep us free from illness.

THE BREATHING PROCESS

Air passes into our lungs through the bronchial tubes. Mucus and cilia in the bronchi and lungs help to keep our lungs clear. They do this by sweeping out any unwanted particles. Oxygen is absorbed into the bloodstream in our lungs, and is then carried by the circulatory system into every cell of our body to help release the

energy stored in the blood. The waste product of this process is carbon dioxide, which is brought back to our lungs and exhaled. We breathe in and out about ten to fifteen times a minute, without having to make a conscious effort. This is enough to blow up several thousand balloons a day.

SMOKING AND POLLUTION

What we breathe becomes a part of us. Cigarette smoke and car fumes are irritants which affect people who suffer from respiratory conditions such as asthma and hayfever. Smoking also contributes to many of the chronic lung conditions, such as lung cancer and emphysema. High

How respiration works

The respiratory system is responsible for introducing oxygen into the blood, which carries it to the tissues, and for removing carbon dioxide from the blood.

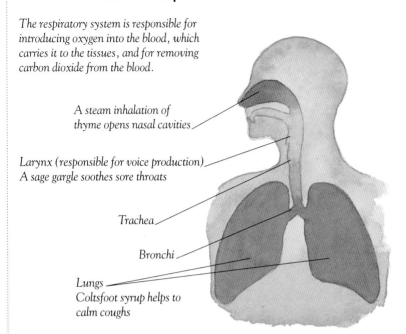

A steam inhalation of thyme opens nasal cavities

Larynx (responsible for voice production)
A sage gargle soothes sore throats

Trachea

Bronchi

Lungs
Coltsfoot syrup helps to calm coughs

levels of pollution in our cities and smoking in the home affect the onset of respiratory diseases in children. There has been an alarming rise in the number of asthmatic children who are dependent on daily doses of steroids in order to breathe.

PREVENTION OF RESPIRATORY DISEASE

Our lifestyle has become more sedentary, and it is now necessary to make an effort to exercise. Our children especially need to be able to run around in the fresh air – something that is becoming more difficult to do with the increase in pollution. Exercise can help to strengthen our lungs. Aerobic exercise forces us to breathe more deeply and fully as the demand for oxygen is increased in the body. Yoga and meditation focus specifically on the way we breathe, helping us to be aware of the expansion and relaxation of the muscles in our chest so that our breathing is less constricted.

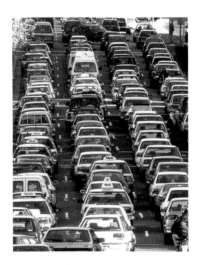

THE CHINESE MEDICINE APPROACH

In Chinese medicine, good, strong, healthy lungs are linked with a strong protective *qi*, or energy. Our lungs help us to fight off viruses and infections before they take hold in the body. The Chinese philosophy is that we receive inspiration through the air we breathe. The lung is related to the metal element, the season of autumn (when a lot of us come down with colds), the color white, and the emotion of grief. An old Chinese saying is that catarrh is unshed tears.

AILMENTS

Ailments affecting the respiratory system are very common. Often these complaints are treated with antibiotics. Herbal remedies can sometimes offer a very effective alternative treatment, especially if they are taken at the first signs of illness. In this section, remedies for

The lungs help to filter the air we breathe, allowing fresh oxygen into the bloodstream and protecting us from pollutants. Higher incidences of asthma and other lung diseases can be related to cigarette smoking and traffic fumes.

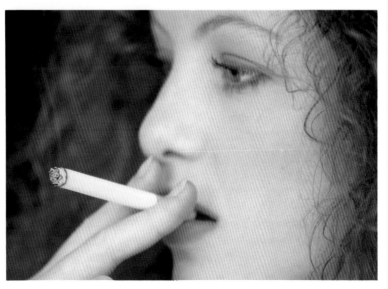

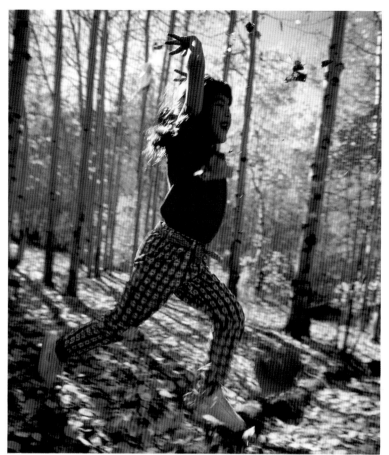

Physical exercise helps to strengthen the body, forcing the lungs to breathe deeply and encouraging the circulation. It plays an important role in a healthy childhood.

The patent remedy *Yin Qiao Jie Du Pien* is famous for getting rid of colds. The two main herbs are *jin yin hua* (honeysuckle) and *lian qiao* (forsythia). These help to clear mild chills and fever, thirst, headache, and cough. It has to be taken with the first signs of a cold, within the first few days of symptoms of sneezing and sore throat, before there is a lot of catarrh. Take one teaspoon of each herb (make sure you use the Chinese herbs) and put them into a teapot with a cup of boiling water. Let it stand for 10 minutes, then drink. Sweeten with honey if desired. Take three times a day.

colds, influenza, sore throats, fevers, sinusitis, tonsilitis, and coughs will be discussed as well as some for asthma and hayfever.

COLDS

Everyone has experienced the common cold. Its symptoms include sneezing, slight chills and fever, scratchy throat, and lots of catarrh. For most people a cold is merely a discomfort; however, the elderly, babies, and asthmatics need to be careful as a common cold could lead to a more serious chest infection. We may catch a cold when we are under stress or rundown and our resistance is low. A cold may be an indication that we need to slow down and rest. A few days off work and some herbal teas can be a very effective treatment!

HERBAL REMEDIES

There are many herbs that are useful in relieving cold symptoms. An infusion of peppermint, elderflower, and yarrow is helpful (*see* Herbal Methods section). Peppermint has a stimulating, decongestant action; elderflower is drying and anticatarrhal; and yarrow is a diaphoretic, helping to clear the virus through a light sweat.

THE CHINESE APPROACH

In Chinese medicine, colds are said to be due to an invasion of wind, cold, or heat. If our defenses are low we are more prone to give in to this invasion. If we are tired and stand in the cold wind, we will end up with a chill, sneezing, and a runny nose. A fever, hot, dry sore throat, and catarrh may follow. When these symptoms appear, the wind and heat have invaded our body.

FEVER

Fever or high body temperature is a natural response to infection. It is the body's way of clearing a virus or bacterial infection through perspiration. As viruses and bacteria are broken down by the cells of the immune system, toxins called pyrogens are released. These cause an increase in the body's metabolism and temperature. They are then sweated out through the skin. A normal body temperature is between 36–37°C (96.8–98.6°F). A fever occurs when the temperature rises above 37.8°C (100°F). If the temperature rises above 38°C (103°F), and does not decrease with tepid sponging down, or if there are signs of convulsions, fits, or stiff neck, consult a doctor immediately.

HERBAL TREATMENT

It is important to drink fluids with a fever to help the body flush out the infection. Try an infusion of camomile or limeflower, which are relaxants as well as diaphoretics. These will help ensure a good sleep, which will speed recovery. Another delicious tea can be made from one teaspoon of grated ginger and one cinnamon stick infused in one cup of boiling water, with some lemon, and honey to taste. This tea encourages sweating and is full of vitamin C, which helps fight infections.

INFLUENZA

If a cold and fever continue over several days, and are accompanied by headache and muscular aches and pains, symptoms of flu have developed. A useful herb for these symptoms is boneset, which will quickly relieve aches and pains, as well as help the body to cope with a fever. It will also help to clear any mucus congestion in the upper respiratory tract, as well as constipation. Use an infusion of the dried or fresh herb. Drink one cup of tea every hour, or as often as possible. Combine boneset with

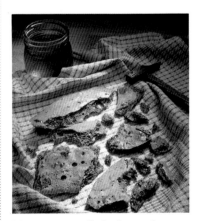

Honey is naturally healing and antiseptic. Add it to your herb tea to soothe sore throats.

elderflower, yarrow, or ginger, depending on your symptoms. Add lemon and honey for flavor, and for vitamin C.

INFLUENZA AND DEPRESSION

If there are signs of depression, which sometimes accompanies influenza, add skullcap to an equal measure of boneset.

SORE THROAT

A sore throat may be the first sign of an infection. If it is accompanied by cold symptoms, use the herbs suggested for colds to help clear the sore throat. A gargle can also be made using a tea of red sage, thyme, or goldenseal. All these herbs have antiseptic properties and will help fight infections. Gargle with these herbs three to six times a day. Just a word of warning: goldenseal is an excellent herb, but it is very bitter and should be used only in small amounts. It should also be avoided during pregnancy.

THE PROTECTIVE ROLE OF THE TONSILS

The tonsils are part of the lymphatic system, and have a protective role in defending the body against infection and pollution. They also act as a filter of poisons in the bloodstream, and those draining from the nose and sinuses. Inflammation of the tonsils indicates an increased fight to rid the body of toxins and infections. Herbal treatment aims at supporting their work, as well as easing the pain, redness, and swelling of tonsillitis.

ACUTE TONSILLITIS

Acute tonsillitis flares up quickly with a painful and red throat. Most

commonly it is a response to a bacterial infection. Use the herbs suggested above for sore throats to ease the discomfort and to soothe the sinus membranes. A gargle of marshmallow tea can soothe a scratchy and burning throat. You should also drink a tea which helps to clear infections: use a mixture of echinacea, calendula, cleavers, and camomile. The echinacea will help to boost the immune system, the calendula and cleavers support the lymphatic tissue in its cleansing work, and the camomile is calming and helps to reduce fevers.

SINUS INFECTIONS

Sinusitis is an infection of the sinus cavities, with symptoms of headache pain and a blocked or runny nose.

HERBAL TREATMENT

For acute sinusitis, use a combination of echinacea to boost the immune system; goldenseal to help clear the catarrh; and marshmallow leaves to soothe the sinus membranes. Avoid goldenseal if you are pregnant. Try substituting one teaspoon of elderflower instead. If there is a fever, add yarrow to the infusion.

STEAM INHALATION

Making a steam inhalation of aromatic herbs such as eucalyptus and pine needles can help to clear the sinuses. Put three teaspoons of leaves in a basin, and add two liters (4 pints) of boiling water. Inhale the steam through the nose for about 10 minutes (*see* Herbal Methods section). Do not go outside immediately after treatment as the mucous membranes will be very sensitive.

A steam inhalation of aromatic herbs, such as pine or eucalyptus, helps to open and clear blocked sinuses.

DIET AND HERBAL TREATMENT

Take a combination of cleavers and calendula as a tincture or tea for a period of several weeks to help clear the sinuses. In cases of chronic sinusitis, it is necessary to look at the diet. An allergy to dairy products may cause an excessive amount of catarrh to be produced, continually inflaming the mucous membranes. Environmental factors, such as dust and pollution, should also be taken into account.

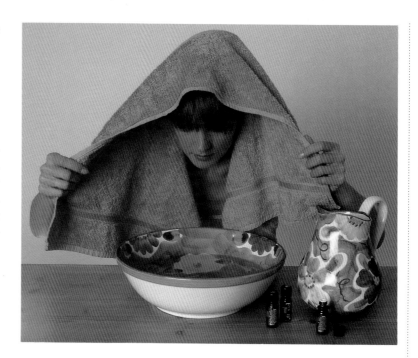

COUGHS

Coughs are the body's attempt to remove obstruction in the throat and chest. Many herbs can be used to clear the throat and chest of irritation, phlegm, and infection, and to build up the immune system. Consult the Herbal Directory and make up a tea from a mixture of herbs to help a particular type of cough.

DRY COUGHS

For a dry, irritating cough, take soothing, moistening herbs such as marshmallow, coltsfoot, and hyssop.

PHLEGMY COUGHS

When the cough has loosened and is producing more phlegm, try a mixture of expectorant herbs such as hyssop, elecampane, and thyme, which should also help to relax the chest and ease coughing spasms. If there is a lot of clear, runny catarrh use ginger and cinnamon to warm and dry it up. A tea of ginger, honey, and lemon will help relieve a cough and cold with chills.

CHEST INFECTIONS

If there are signs of a chest infection, such as fever, pain with coughing, and green phlegm, use a combination of echinacea with either elderflower, yarrow, or limeflower. If fever is persistently high or breathing is difficult, seek professional medical help.

ASTHMA

Over the last decade there has been a dramatic rise in diagnosed cases of asthma. Many people treat their asthma successfully by using steroid inhalers. Herbal treatment can be used alongside other medication to help reduce the need for these drugs, and to prevent the onset of colds and coughs, which can aggravate asthma attacks. Herbal treatment needs to take place over several months to be effective. Any reduction in medication should be done only with professional medical advice.

THE DIET FACTOR

Asthma attacks can be triggered by allergic reactions to foods. The most common food allergens are milk produce, wheat, oranges, eggs, artificial colorings, and preservatives (especially sulphur). Avoid eating one of these foods for several weeks and note if there is any difference in the number of attacks, breathlessness, or general vitality.

ENVIRONMENTAL FACTORS

The house dustmite is another strong factor in asthma, and is prevalent in modern homes with central heating and carpets. Pets and animals can also be a trigger of wheezing and asthma attacks.

HERBAL TREATMENT

There are a number of herbal prescriptions for asthma, and you should seek professional help from a herbalist. For mild cases, the following herbs will be effective, especially if taken over a period of months: echinacea, borage, and licorice will all support the immune system and adrenal glands, which are often low in asthmatics.

Combine one of these with coltsfoot, hyssop, elecampane, and thyme. These four herbs together will help to clear the phlegm and strengthen the lungs. If stress and tension are around, add either skullcap, vervain, or camomile. These are relaxants, which may help the breathing to become slower and deeper.

CHINESE HERBAL TREATMENT

Chinese herbal medicine has much to offer in the treatment of asthma. There is not enough space here to mention the dried herbs used, but *ma huang* is especially effective for attacks. This herb should only be used under the guidance of a herbalist. The patent remedy *Qing Qi Hua Tan Wan* (Clean Air Tea) is used when there is phlegm that feels stuck in the chest, causing wheeziness. It can help to move the phlegm and open the chest. The formula *Sang Ju Yin* is useful to treat the first symptoms of a cold that goes straight on to the chest.

HAYFEVER

H ayfever is an allergic reaction to the various plant pollens. It is best to start treatment a few months before the hayfever season. Taking daily decoctions of echinacea or ginseng can help to build up the immune system and prevent allergic responses. Another interesting treatment is to take a dessertspoonful of honey with the honeycomb with each meal for a month before the season begins. Continue throughout the spring and summer.

TREATING SYMPTOMS

Once the allergic reactions begin, a combination of elderflower, eyebright, and camomile can be added to the treatment. The elderflower helps to dry the catarrh, the eyebright strengthens the eyes, and the camomile soothes the inflammation.

CHINESE HERBAL TREATMENT

An excellent Chinese herbal remedy is the patent formula *Bi Yan Pian*. This formula helps to clear the nose, stop sneezing, cool and soothe the eyes, and remove heat caused by the inflammation of the mucous membranes.

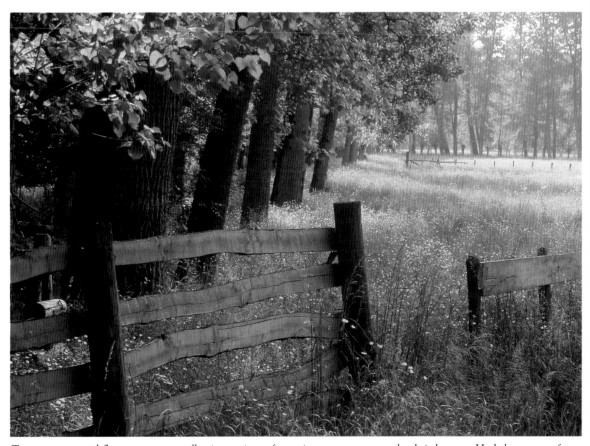

Trees, grasses, and flowers can cause allergic reactions of sneezing, runny nose, and red, itchy eyes. Herbal treatment for these symptoms of hayfever can be very effective.

THE EYES AND EARS

Sight and hearing, along with the other senses of taste, touch, and smell,

help us to perceive, understand, and survive in the world around us.

AILMENTS OF THE EYES AND EARS

Many eye and ear problems can be helped by herbal treatment, especially if diagnosed early. Herbal treatment is gentle yet effective for acute complaints such as conjunctivitis, styes, ear infections, and earache. Chronic eye conditions, glue ear, and tinnitus require long-term treatment, but also may respond well to herbs.

CONJUNCTIVITIS AND BLEPHARITIS

In conjunctivitis the eye becomes irritated because of an infection, an allergy such as hayfever, or pollution. Blepharitis is a more serious condition in which the eyelids become red and inflamed. Take a mixture of echinacea and eyebright as a tea three times a day or as pills

to help boost immunity and detoxify the system. If the conjunctivitis is due to allergies, drink a tea of eyebright, camomile, and yarrow three times a day. To ease inflammation, place wet camomile teabags on closed eyes for 10 minutes.

AN HERBAL EYEWASH

Bathe the eyes regularly using an eyewash of eyebright tea. Make sure you use a sterilized eyebath and a separate solution and towel for each eye, as these conditions are highly contagious.

A HELPFUL CHINESE HERBAL TEA

The Chinese herb *ju hua* is also very effective in relieving symptoms of dry, red eyes with a sensitivity to light. *Ju hua* or chrysanthemum tea can be drunk regularly to help the eyes, as well as some headaches.

STYES

Styes are infections at the base of the eyelashes. They are usually an indication of being tired or run-down. They are highly contagious, so it is important to use separate towels when washing. Apply warm compresses (*see* Herbal Methods section) of eyebright, burdock, or calendula tea frequently throughout the day until the stye bursts or is reabsorbed by the body. Take echinacea, garlic, or goldenseal to help clear the infection.

CHRONIC EYE CONDITIONS

Chronic eye conditions such as glaucoma, cataracts, and macular degeneration need long-term treatment under professional medical

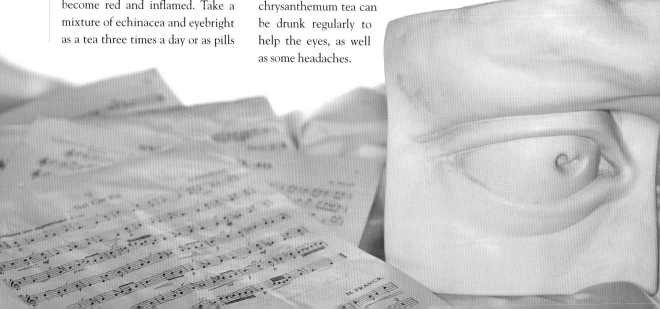

How the eyes and ears work

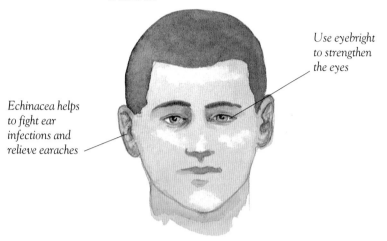

Sight and hearing, along with the other senses of taste, touch, and smell, help us to perceive and understand the world around us.

Use eyebright to strengthen the eyes

Echinacea helps to fight ear infections and relieve earaches

supervision. Herbal treatment, as well as advice on vitamins and minerals, can help prevent and slow down deterioration. Antioxidants and bilberry will help to slow down macular degeneration and increase visual acuity.

CHINESE REMEDIES

Two well-known Chinese patent formulae that are useful are *Qi Ju Di Huang Wan* and *Ming Mu Di Huang Wan*. They are good for chronic conditions (*see* Chinese Patent Remedies). Do not stop any medication prescribed by your doctor without his consent; the herbs are to be used as supplements only.

EAR INFECTIONS

Infections of the ear often start in the throat and spread through the Eustachian tube. Herbal remedies that are antimicrobial and anticatarrhal such as goldenseal and echinacea should be taken as a pill, tea, or tincture. Garlic should be added to food or taken as garlic perles. For external use, first warm the garlic perle in your hands, then place a few drops of garlic oil from a perle in the ear, providing there is

no skin irritation in the ear canal. Keep the oil in with a cotton plug.

EARACHE

Relieve the pain of an ear infection with a few drops of warm mullein oil or almond oil, or a few drops from a strong infusion of camomile, yarrow, or hyssop tea. If there is much pain, a high fever, or thick discharge, call a doctor immediately.

GLUE EAR

Chronic ear infections can result in a condition whereby the hearing is diminished by wax and catarrh stuck in the middle ear. Lymphatic tonics such as cleavers and calendula need to be used with herbs like elderflower, goldenseal, and hyssop, which help to clear catarrh. Treatment may need to be over several months. For children, tinctures are often easier to give. A dairy-free diet may need to be tried for several weeks, as dairy products often cause the body to produce more mucus.

TINNITUS

Tinnitus creates the symptom of noises in the ear. Regular use of goldenseal or black cohosh taken over a period of time may help. The Chinese patent remedy *Lui Wei Di Huang Wan* may help, especially with the elderly. A variation called *Er Ming Zuo Ci Wan* may help if the tinnitus is related to high blood pressure. Ginkgo will help to decrease tinnitus for most people but it needs to be taken for up to three months for results to be felt.

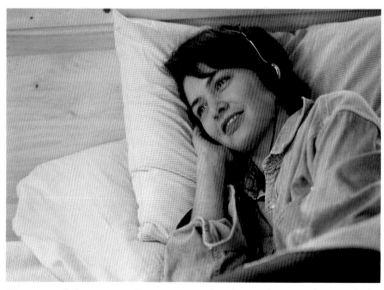

Tinnitus and chronic ear infections can result in hearing loss, interfering with the pleasure of hearing sounds around us. Herbal remedies can be helpful in the treatment of these conditions.

THE DIGESTIVE SYSTEM

Our health and vitality depends on eating a well-balanced diet and the functioning of an efficient digestive system. Absorption of essential nutrients supplies the body with the necessary building blocks to keep it fit and strong.

The digestive system begins in the mouth, where food is chewed and mixed with enzymes in the saliva to break it down. It passes through the esophagus to the stomach. Here, food is partly digested through the action of more enzymes, and strong acid secretions which kill any harmful bacteria. In the small intestine or duodenum, the food is mixed with enzyme-rich secretions from the pancreas and gut wall, and with bile from the liver. Essential nutrients are absorbed into the bloodstream and taken to the liver, where they are processed. In the large intestine or colon, the fluids are absorbed into the bloodstream, leaving the residue, or fecal matter, to be expelled.

INTERACTION WITH THE BODY

A good digestive system is a key factor in maintaining health and well-being. If the digestive system is weak or upset, we can feel tired, irritable, and be unable to concentrate and sleep. If elimination through the bowel is upset, essential food nutrients can be lost, for example in cases of duodenal ulcers and chronic diarrhea. Constipation can give rise to many other complaints, such as low immunity and headaches, due to toxins not being evacuated.

THE CHINESE MEDICINE APPROACH

In Chinese medicine digestion plays an important role in the good health of the body. The stomach and spleen are the main organs related to the digestive system, and they have the functions of breaking down the food and transporting nutrients throughout the body. They have a vital part in the production of *qi*, or energy. The protective *qi*, or *wei qi*, which is the basis for our immune system, is dependent on strong digestion. It is interesting that recent scientific investigations have found a strong correlation between a good immunity system and a healthy digestive system.

PREVENTION OF DIGESTIVE DISORDERS

Many disorders of the digestive system can be helped by a careful diet and good eating habits. Meals should be eaten regularly, with breakfast being as important as other meals. Meal times should be relaxed. Time should be allowed to chew food properly, and to allow it to be digested. The diet should include fresh fruit, vegetables, and natural cereals to provide nutrients and roughage. Sugar, starches, and refined flour should be kept to a minimum, and artificial additives should be avoided. Coffee, tea, alcohol, and smoking should also be restricted as they upset the digestive system.

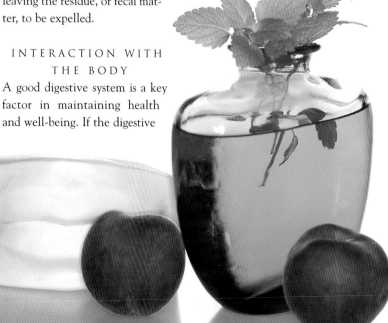

CONSTIPATION

Food is broken down into a few simple forms which the body is able to utilize to provide the raw materials and energy for cellular activity.

Food is reduced to a semi-fluid mass in the mouth

Food is stored in the stomach. A gruel of slippery elm powder softens the effects of acid indigestion

Food is broken down into simple compounds by the digestive juices of the gut, pancreas, and liver

Dandelion is an excellent liver tonic and cleanser

The broken down food is absorbed into the bloodstream via the small intestines

Excess water in the residue is removed in the largel intestines. The Chinese patent remedy Shen Ling Bai Zhu Pian *is very helpful for chronic diarrhea*

The feces are excreted through the anus

Eating too much refined food and not enough fruits, vegetables, and wholegrains, which contain roughage, is a major cause of constipation. Lack of exercise, stress, and food allergies can also result in constipation. In chronic constipation, the muscles of the bowel need to be stimulated to push the stools out. Long-term use of laxatives can block this natural movement (peristalsis). With aging, the bowel can become weak and sluggish, needing more roughage and moisture to help the contents move through smoothly.

HERBAL TREATMENT

Gentle remedies like linseed and psyllium seeds can help to provide bulk and roughage. Soak one or two teaspoons of these seeds in 200 ml (8 fl oz) of hot water for two hours. Add lemon and honey for flavor, and drink before bedtime. If needed, another drink can be taken first thing in the morning as well. Linseed can also be added to a bowl of wholegrain cereal for breakfast. A decoction of more stimulating laxative herbs can be taken for up to two weeks. Use a combination of licorice, dandelion root, yellow dockroot, burdock, and ginger. If

THE EFFECT OF STRESS AND TENSION

The digestive system is richly supplied with nerves, making it prone to the effects of stress and nervous tension. The autonomic nervous system regulates the blood supply to and from the digestive system, as well as the production of the digestive juices. The digestive system is susceptible to our thoughts and emotions, and we use the phrase "gut reaction."

AILMENTS

In this section, ailments relating to the whole system, such as constipation, diarrhea, nausea and vomiting, and gastric pain will be discussed. The digestive system will then be divided into its parts, so

that ailments relating more specifically to the mouth, stomach, small intestines, and large intestines are reviewed. Herbal treatment, along with some dietary advice, will be suggested for each ailment.

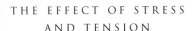

A healthy diet of fresh foods including fruits and vegetables will provide nutrients and roughage. Good eating habits are important to help maintain a strong digestive system.

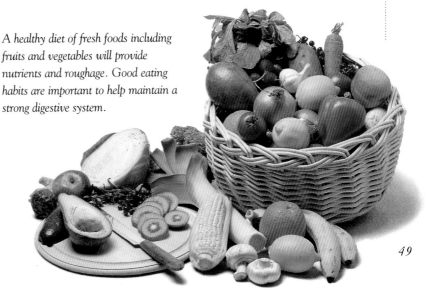

stress and tension are involved, add camomile or crampbark. If constipation persists or is painful, seek professional medical advice.

DIARRHEA

Acute diarrhea is the body's way of eliminating poisons or infections. It can occur with food poisoning or stomach bugs. For mild diarrhea, drink a tea of meadowsweet to soothe and calm the gut. If it is related to an infection, drink teas of camomile, thyme, ginger, or fennel, either on their own or in combination to help fight the infection and relieve ache and discomfort. Sometimes bouts of diarrhea can be due to tension. In this case, drink teas of camomile or lemon balm combined with meadowsweet to help relax the gut. If diarrhea persists, or if there is blood or mucus in the stools, seek professional medical advice.

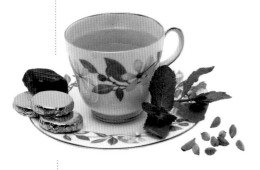

Teas and tinctures made from a combination of herbs are a gentle but effective way of easing the discomfort of digestive complaints.

A CHINESE REMEDY
The Chinese patent remedy *Shen Ling Bai Zhu Pian* is excellent for chronic diarrhea due to weakness in the digestive system. It helps to tone digestion, and relieve symptoms of belching, bloating, indiges-tion, and abdominal fullness, as well as loose stools. It can be used with children, and is especially helpful to those who are fussy eaters, or who have allergic reactions to food. It can be used for prolonged periods.

NAUSEA AND VOMITING

Nausea and vomiting can be symptoms of food poisoning, stomach infections, morning sickness, migraine, or nervousness. To help settle the stomach, sip teas of ginger root, peppermint, or camomile. As they all have their own flavor, choose one that suits your individual taste; add honey if preferred. If there is an infection, add tinctures of echinacea or goldenseal to teas of lavender, thyme, or lemon balm. If stress is involved, drink teas of camomile, lemon balm, or passion flower to help relax. If vomiting is severe or persistent, call the doctor immediately.

DIGESTIVE PAINS
Pain in the digestive system can be symptomatic of different problems. Any strong or persistent pains should be investigated by a doctor. Colic and griping pains are usually due to muscle spasms in the gut as it attempts to push its contents through the system. Carminative herbs, such as peppermint, ginger, fennel, lemon balm, and camomile, which are specific for relieving gas and wind, can be taken as a tea or tincture in warm water after meals. Add warming spices, such as cinnamon, ginger, and cardamom to foods to ease the digestion. Massage the abdomen in a clockwise direction with a few drops of warming oils of cinnamon, ginger, cloves, or peppermint diluted in a base oil.

THE MOUTH

The digestive system begins in the mouth. Problems with the teeth and gums can make the chewing of food difficult. Treatments for toothache, gingivitis, abscesses, and mouth ulcers will be suggested below, enabling the whole digestive process to be more efficient. Dental hygiene is an important part of preventative care.

TOOTHACHE
When problems arise, teeth must be treated by a dentist. A herbal first-aid remedy for toothache is to chew some cloves, which contain a pain-relieving oil called eugenol. Alternatively, soak a piece of cotton (cotton wool) in clove oil and place it next to the tooth. Peppermint oil can be used in the same way, but is not as effective.

GINGIVITIS
Gingivitis is an infection of the superficial tissue of the gum. It can cause the gums to appear red and swollen and to bleed easily. Much of gum disease can be reduced through good oral hygiene and by avoiding sugars and refined, processed foods. Take garlic or echinacea to help fight infections. Rinse the mouth with a teaspoon of a mixture of echinacea and myrrh tinctures in a small amount of water. This does not have a pleasant taste, but is very effective.

ABSCESSES
A tooth abscess is a very painful condition that must be seen by the dentist. Antibiotics are the conventional form of treatment, and are usually quite effective. A herbal remedy can be made from a decoction of echinacea, cleavers, and poke root, which will help to

A bright smile with healthy gums and teeth is a vital part of our expression. Good dental hygiene reduces the risk of toothache and gum infections.

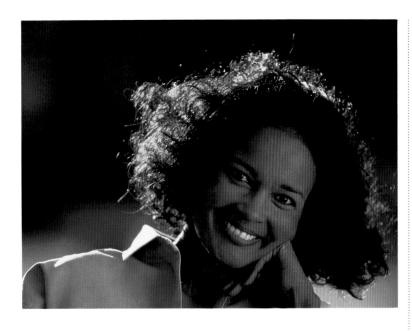

fight the infection and cleanse the lymphatic system. Garlic perles and high doses of vitamin C are also beneficial.

MOUTH ULCERS

Mouth ulcers can indicate that the body is run down or under stress. Recovery from colds and flu, or the use of antibiotics and stress can cause an outbreak of mouth ulcers. The whole body should be treated with strengthening and calming teas of ginseng, lemon balm, vervain, and licorice. Coffee, tea, and cigarette smoking should be avoided. Treat the ulcers with a mouthwash of red sage and myrrh. In North America a commercially-produced licorice extract called "deglycyrrhizinated licorice," or "DGL," is also used in the treatment of ulcers and hyperacidity (*see* page 122).

THE STOMACH

The main function of the stomach is to digest food by mixing it with digestive enzymes and hydrochloric acid. Stomach acid helps to break down the food and sterilize it so that harmful bacteria are not passed on.

INDIGESTION

Symptoms of indigestion can vary from pain and heartburn to discomfort and flatulence. They are often triggered by stress and excitement, irregular meals, and over-eating. Foods that are rich, fatty, or spicy should be avoided as well as coffee, tea, cigarettes, and alcohol. Being allergic to certain foods will also bring on symptoms of indigestion. The underlying cause of the indigestion needs to be treated; a change in diet and lifestyle may be what is required to bring about a long-term cure.

HERBAL TREATMENT

With the first sign of discomfort, take slippery elm powder or tablets to soothe the inflamed stomach lining. Drink teas made from a mixture of meadowsweet, marshmallow, and licorice, which will help to reduce stomach acid and heal inflammation. After meals, drink teas of camomile, rosemary, peppermint, and fennel to help settle the stomach and aid digestion. If stress and tension are around, drink teas of camomile, lemon balm, and vervain to aid relaxation.

GASTRITIS

Gastritis is an irritation of the stomach lining, which can be caused by an infection or a reaction to food. It can start with an acute case of food poisoning or a stomach bug, and last for a while afterward. The treatment for gastritis is through diet and herbs. Drinks such as coffee, tea, and alcohol, and rich, spicy, and greasy foods should be avoided. With acute inflammation do not eat foods high in fiber or acid, such as bran, nuts, seeds, tomatoes, vinegar, and pickles. Do not smoke, as this increases the production of stomach acid.

HERBAL TREATMENT

A decoction of the following herbs will help to soothe and heal the stomach lining. Use a mixture of one part marshmallow root and meadowsweet to one half-part goldenseal. The goldenseal has a powerful healing quality for the membranes of the stomach lining, but as it also stimulates the muscles of the uterus, it should be avoided during pregnancy. If stress and tension are aggravating the gastritis, add valerian to the decoction. Drink this tea after each meal until the condition clears.

GASTRIC ULCER

A gastric ulcer occurs when the mucous membranes of the stomach lining break down and the digestive juices start to irritate the stomach wall. Herbal treatment is similar to gastritis. Take a decoction of marshmallow root, meadowsweet, and goldenseal. The marshmallow

51

root is soothing and healing to the stomach membranes. The meadowsweet helps to settle the stomach and slow the production of acid. The goldenseal is beneficial to the mucous membranes, but should be avoided in pregnancy. Take slippery elm as a powder or tablet morning and night to help protect the stomach from acid.

FOODS TO AVOID

If a gastric ulcer forms, it is an indication that changes in the diet and lifestyle are needed if the ulcer is to clear permanently. The diet should be low in fiber and protein while the ulcer pain is acute. Eat small, well-cooked meals of easily digestible foods frequently. Avoid alcohol, tea, coffee, and tobacco as well as acidic, spicy, or greasy foods. As the ulcer heals, eat a well-balanced diet, reintroducing fiber and proteins. It is best to seek professional advice for this condition.

A CHINESE REMEDY

Bu Zhong Yi Qi Wan is a Chinese patent remedy that helps to strengthen the digestive system. It should not be used with acute conditions, but with more chronic complaints of abdominal bloating, pain, flatulence, and erratic stools. It contains herbs which strengthen the digestion such as astralagus (*huang qi*), licorice (*gan cao*), and ginger root (*sheng jiang*). It also contains herbs that help move the digestive *qi*, or energy, so that feelings of fullness and abdominal bloating are eased.

THE INTESTINES

The small intestine makes up the longest part of the digestive system—its length can be up to 60 meters (20 feet). Its main function is to absorb nutrients from the food into the bloodstream. The large intestine absorbs water and minerals. Bacteria in the gut (gut flora) help to make vitamins and to clear toxic bacteria.

DUODENAL ULCERS

The duodenum is the first part of the small intestines. It starts below the pyloric sphincter, which is the valve that separates the stomach and small intestines. If it does not function properly, acid from the stomach leaks into the alkaline environment of the small intestines and can cause an ulcer.

HERBAL TREATMENT

Make a decoction of marshmallow and licorice root with meadowsweet and goldenseal to help heal and soothe the damaged lining. Always refer to the contraindications in the Herbal Directory before using goldenseal, licorice, or any other herb. Drink this before meals. Slippery elm powder taken as a gruel will help to coat the gut lining and protect it from acidity and irritation. Take this first thing in the morning and last thing at night. Eat little and often, and avoid spicy, fatty, or greasy foods, vinegar, coffee, tea, alcohol, and tobacco. It is best to seek professional advice for treatment for this condition.

STRESS AND TENSION

For feelings of stress and tension that often accompany ulcers, drink relaxing teas of camomile, lemon balm, vervain, and skullcap, which will help to strengthen the nervous system and ease tension. Take an herbal bath with oils or strong infusions of lavender, camomile, and lemon balm.

IRRITABLE BOWEL SYNDROME (IBS)

The workings of the bowel are susceptible to our emotions. Stress and tension, along with poor eating habits and food intolerances, can aggravate any inflammation and irritation in the lining of the bowel. Symptoms of IBS include alternating diarrhea and constipation, flatulence, and griping pains. This can vary from

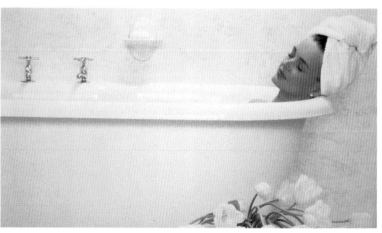

An herbal bath with strong infusions of lavender, camomile, and lemon balm will help to relieve stress that may aggravate digestive complaints. Take a relaxing bath to soothe away cares and tensions.

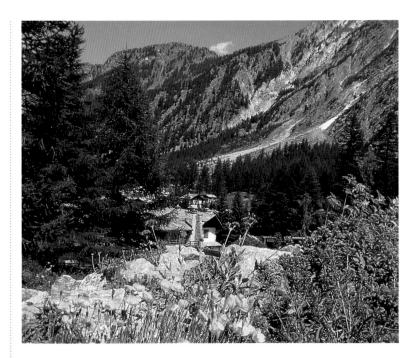

Herbal folklore suggests a "spring tonic" to cleanse and revitalize the body after a winter lacking in physical exercise and fresh foods. This tonic often included herbs which supported the liver.

discomfort to severe pain with diarrhea. Eliminating any suspected food allergies can do a lot to relieve symptoms. Most common ones include tea, coffee, milk, eggs, wheat, or gluten. Any severe pain, or persistent diarrhea or constipation, needs medical attention.

HERBAL TREATMENT
Drink a tea made from a combination of wild yam, camomile, peppermint, marshmallow, and goldenseal. The wild yam will help to relieve spasms; the camomile and peppermint will encourage good digestion; the marshmallow will soothe the inflammation; and the goldenseal helps to heal the membranes (but should only be used in small doses, and not if pregnant). Drink this three times a day over a period of time. Instead of coffee and tea, drink simple herbal teas of camomile, lemon balm, and fennel to help relax and ease tensions.

A CHINESE REMEDY
The Chinese patent formula *Xiao Yao Wan* (Free and Easy Wanderer) is helpful in cases of IBS, especially if it is worse during times of stress and accompanies PMT. It helps to relax the *qi*, or energy, and encourages digestion. It is useful with symptoms of abdominal bloating, fullness, and poor appetite, and those symptoms which are related to food allergies.

HEMORRHOIDS
Hemorrhoids, or piles, is a painful condition related to the blood vessels of the rectum and anus. The most common cause is chronic constipation, and if this can be avoided, the piles will be relieved. A simple infusion of the herb pilewort may tone the vessels and ease their inflammation. The astringent qualities of witch hazel, which can be made into a suppository (*see* Herbal Methods section), will also help to shrink and relieve pain.

THE LIVER AND GALLBLADDER

The liver is the largest organ inside the body, and plays a vital role in the digestive process. It is involved in the processing of carbohydrates and is the most important organ in maintaining blood sugar levels. It helps to break down proteins and fats. It stores vitamins A, D, K, and B12. The fat-soluble vitamins depend on bile, which is produced in the liver, for their absorption. The liver also helps to regulate hormones. It detoxifies drugs and other chemicals; helping to keep the body clear and well-functioning. The liver produces and secretes bile, which is stored in the gallbladder. Bile helps to break down and absorb fats, as well as activate the pancreas.

HERBAL TREATMENT FOR THE LIVER
Spring tonics are part of folk remedy tradition, and are used to cleanse and support the liver after a winter of bad food. They are still relevant for the stresses of modern life. Pollution, food additives, greasy fast foods, and drug and alcohol abuse all put strain on the liver. A useful liver tonic can be made from dandelion, meadowsweet, and goldenseal. The roots and leaves of dandelion make a good tonic and cleanser for the liver and the kidneys; meadowsweet will support the stomach; and goldenseal (use in small doses and avoid if pregnant) helps to tone and stimulate the digestive system. Milk thistle is another excellent herb which supports and helps to cleanse the liver. Drink two liters (4 pints) of water a day to flush the system, and avoid eating any fried, roasted, or fatty foods.

THE URINARY SYSTEM

The urinary system has the important task of regulating the amount of water in the body and producing urine to carry away waste products. Its functioning is vital to keeping the body healthy and fit by preventing dehydration and a buildup of toxic material.

The kidneys and bladder are the two main organs of the urinary system. The kidneys work to regulate water in the body, filter and cleanse the blood, and restore body fluids to a pure and useful state. Waste is passed out through the urine, which leaves the kidneys via the ureter to the bladder, where it is stored. It is then discharged out of the body through the urethra.

AILMENTS

In this section herbal treatment for discomforts such as cystitis and urethritis will be discussed, as well as other related problems, such as water retention and incontinence. More serious conditions, such as prostate and kidney problems, may need advice from a professional herbalist, but some supportive herbal treatments will be suggested.

THE KIDNEYS

The renal artery brings circulating blood to the kidneys for filtering. This is a complex process, which involves the absorption of essential nutrients, cleansing of wastes, and reabsorption of nutrients back into the body. The kidneys also help maintain the acid-alkaline balance of the blood, and regulate the salt balance within the body. The adrenal glands, which produce adrenaline, are situated on top of the kidneys. They can affect the kidneys' secretion of sodium into the blood, and the production of the hormone renin.

THE CHINESE MEDICINE APPROACH

In Chinese medicine there is a strong link between the kidney and the bladder. They are related to our energy reserves, which are frequently depleted in our society where there is a strong emphasis on achievement and hard work. The season associated with the water element, which is related to the kidney and bladder, is winter. This is the time for resting and replenishing energy so that there will be a strong start to new growth in the spring. Weak kidney and bladder *qi*, or energy, can be related to many complaints of low-back ache and fatigue, as well as the ailments listed here.

Nitrogenous wastes (mainly as the simple compound urea) and acids are removed from the blood by the kidneys.

Blood in

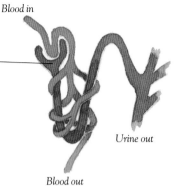

Tubules
The fluid part of the blood (free of cells and protein) is filtered under pressure into long tubules in the kidney. The tubules are selectively permeable, and most of the fluid and any essential compounds are reabsorbed back into the blood. For kidney infections, drink an herbal tea of echinacea, celery seed, couchgrass, and yarrow

Urine
A small fraction of the fluid containing waste matter remains in the tubules and forms the urine

Urine out

Blood out

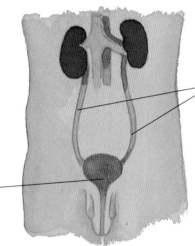

The ureters
The urine passes down the ureters. Barley water helps to alkalize the urine and ease burning pains of cystitis and urethritis

The bladder
From the ureters the urine passes into the bladder and is excreted at intervals. Drink a tea of marshmallow, couchgrass, and yarrow to soothe bladder inflammation

PREVENTION OF AILMENTS

Healthy functioning of any part of the body relies on the kidneys' ability to eliminate waste products and toxins. Our food and diet tend to contain many chemicals and artificial products, which puts a strain on kidney function. It is important to drink plenty of liquids to help the kidneys flush through toxins and prevent illness. Avoid drinking excessive amounts of alcohol, coffee, and tea to make their job easier. To prevent strain on the bladder, try to pass water when the urge is felt rather than holding out for long periods.

CYSTITIS AND URETHRITIS

Infection of the bladder or urethra can be a chronic or acute condition. Symptoms include a burning pain on passing urine, often accompanied by pain in the groin during or just after urination. A desire to pass water although the bladder is empty is another common symptom. Drink plenty of water to help clear the infection. Cranberry juice or extract will also help by preventing the bacteria's ability to adhere to the wall of the bladder. Take a tea of marshmallow,

couchgrass, and yarrow to soothe the inflammation. If it is at the early stage, which is the best time to treat cystitis, an infusion of yarrow tea drunk three times a day may solve the problem. You can add camomile to help relax if feelings of anxiety and tension are present. If the burning is very strong, cornsilk may be added. If pain is severe, or there is a fever, seek professional medical help.

A SOOTHING DRINK

To help alkalize the urine and ease some of the burning, drink barley water throughout the day. Use 100 g (4 oz) of washed barley with 600 ml

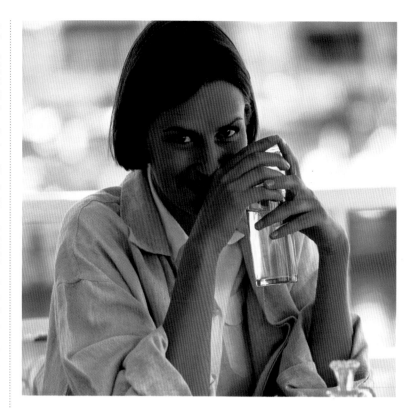

Drink plenty of liquid each day to help support the kidneys' function of clearing the toxins out of the body.

day (*see* Herbal Methods section). For a swollen prostate gland, take a zinc supplement, or eat a handful of pumpkin seeds daily. A teaspoonful of safflower oil or cold-pressed linseed oil daily will help supply essential fatty acids. Drink a decoction of false unicorn root, dandelion, saw palmetto, couchgrass, and prickly ash three times a day. Take plenty of exercise. Any swelling or discomfort of the prostate should be investigated by a doctor.

WATER RETENTION

Water retention can be a symptom of many different problems, from circulation and kidney complaints to hormonal imbalance. It is important to find the cause of the problem, and this may involve medical tests. To treat cases of mild water retention, drink any herbal teas which have diuretic properties, the best ones being dandelion leaf and yarrow. (*See* Herbal Directory, page 142 for more information on the diuretic powers of dandelion.) If there is no improvement in 10 days, seek medical attention. If the water retention is part of premenstrual symptoms, add *vitex* to help balance the hormones.

INCONTINENCE

Incontinence has both physical and psychological causes. If there is no major physical defect, herbal treatment may be helpful. It is worth a try in cases where

(1 pint) water. Simmer in a nonaluminum pot with a lid until the barley is soft. Strain and keep the liquid. Add a small amount of honey and lemon, and drink this warm.

PREVENTION
Some women are prone to urinary-tract infection. Any disturbance within the body may start off an attack of cystitis or urethritis. Stress, overwork, and antibiotics may lower resistance to infection. In this case it is important to drink at least 1 liter (2 pints) of water daily and urinate frequently. Avoid coffee, sugar, and acidic foods such as tomatoes and citrus fruits. In some individuals, caffeine will prevent the bladder from completely emptying. Deodorant douches and bathing in soapy water may cause irritation, and should be avoided.

A CHINESE HERBAL REMEDY
There are many useful Chinese herbal remedies for cystitis and urethritis. The remedies vary, depending on whether the symptoms include blood in the urine, cloudy urine, acute pain, or chronic discomfort. *Bu Zhong Yi Qi Wan* is a patent remedy useful in cases of the more chronic type. Symptoms include difficult urination that comes in a weak stream, slight abdominal distension, and general tiredness. This remedy is a general tonic that helps to raise the *qi*, or energy, allowing the infection to clear from the body.

PROSTATITIS

An infection of the prostate gland is generally not as localized as cystitis, and may need a more overall approach. Echinacea is a good herbal antibiotic, and should be combined with couchgrass, celery seed, and horsetail. Add saw palmetto as a tonic for the male hormone and gland; it helps to shrink the prostate gland. Take as a decoction or tincture three times a incontinence is due to a loss of tone of the sphincter muscle, or to general muscle or nervous debility. Make a decoction of two parts horsetail and one part agrimony, and drink this three times a day (*see* Herbal Methods section).

BEDWETTING

A child over the age of six who still wets the bed regularly may need medical investigation to see if there is an underlying physical problem. Bedwetting can also be due to stress, anxiety, and food allergies. Avoid giving drinks before bed, take the child to the toilet in the night, and try to encourage dry nights with small rewards. A tea made from St John's wort, horsetail, and cornsilk sweetened with honey, will help to soothe any irritation in the bladder. Add camomile, skullcap, or lemon balm if the child is stressed or worried.

A CHINESE HERB
The Chinese herbal repertory consists mainly of plants; however, it also uses some animal parts, and even stones and minerals. For example, the Chinese herb chicken livers (*ji nei jin*) is a useful remedy for bedwetting in children. It is very effective and easy to give. The chicken livers come as a powder, which can be mixed into juice or water. Use 2 g (1 tsp) powder daily for several weeks. The remedy can also help with incontinence in adults, and to dissolve urinary stones—but professional advice is needed for both problems.

KIDNEY STONES

The formation of stones, or mineral deposits, in the kidney responds well to herbal treatment. A low-acid diet is recommended to help stop the stones forming; this means totally avoiding foods high in oxalic acid, such as rhubarb and spinach. Drink up to 3 liters (6 pints) of water a day, preferably one with a low mineral content, to help flush out the system. Take a combination of herbs as tea or tinctures to help dissolve and wash out the stones or gravel. A mixture of couchgrass, dandelion leaves, cleavers, marshmallow, and stone root will help this condition. Extra vitamin B6 and magnesium will prevent new stones forming.

KIDNEY INFECTIONS

Kidney infections are a serious and painful condition, and need professional medical advice. The herbal treatment suggested here can be used to support medical treatment. Drink plenty of liquids, avoiding coffee, tea, and alcohol. Instead, drink camomile and lime-blossom tea to help relax and ease pain. Take a mixture of echinacea, celery seed, couchgrass, and yarrow to help fight the infection. Drink 600 ml (1 pint) of tea a day.

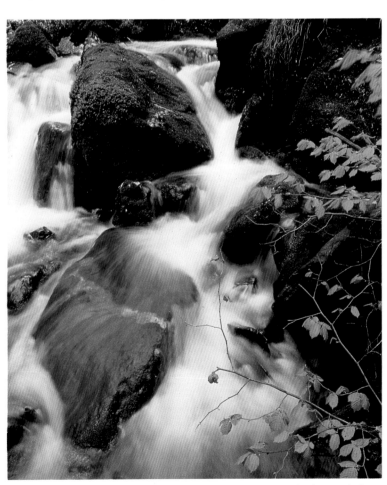

A large part of our body is water. Drinking one liter (two pints) of water daily will help to maintain a well-functioning urinary system.

THE REPRODUCTIVE SYSTEM

The reproductive system is one of nature's most miraculous "inventions,"

yet it also can cause anguish, pain, and discomfort if there are problems.

Primarily the female reproductive system is discussed here, along with

some suggestions for herbs to help male impotence and low sperm count.

The primary female reproductive organs are the ovaries, which secrete the hormones progesterone and estrogen and produce the ova, or eggs. Hormones secreted by the pituitary gland interact with those released by the ovaries to create the menstrual cycle. Ovulation occurs about 14 days into the menstrual cycle. If fertilization occurs, pregnancy begins. If the egg is not fertilized, it is shed with the lining of the uterus at the end of the 28-day cycle.

CHANGES IN THE MENSTRUAL CYCLE

From the onset of the menses through to menopause the menstrual cycle varies with each woman. Hormonal changes due to pregnancy and birth, aging, and life events all affect the menstrual cycle. For some women this is not a problem, yet others may need some support for the discomforts brought on by these hormonal changes. Herbal treatment has been used by women for many centuries to help the body to cope with these changes.

NATIVE AMERICAN TRADITIONS

In Native American tradition, there is a strong relationship with the earth as the mother who looks after us, providing food and a home. Traditionally herbs were seen as part of the earth's gifts. Herb gathering was always done with prayers of thanks, and some of the plant

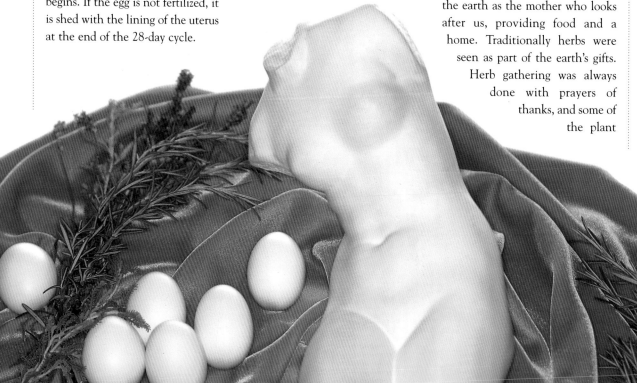

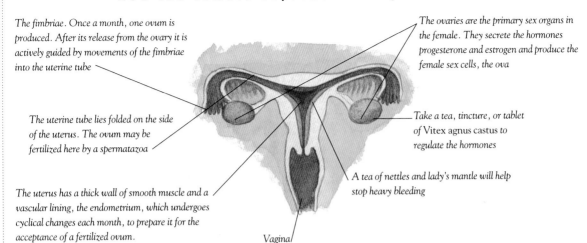

The fimbriae. Once a month, one ovum is produced. After its release from the ovary it is actively guided by movements of the fimbriae into the uterine tube

The ovaries are the primary sex organs in the female. They secrete the hormones progesterone and estrogen and produce the female sex cells, the ova

The uterine tube lies folded on the side of the uterus. The ovum may be fertilized here by a spermatazoa

Take a tea, tincture, or tablet of Vitex agnus castus to regulate the hormones

The uterus has a thick wall of smooth muscle and a vascular lining, the endometrium, which undergoes cyclical changes each month, to prepare it for the acceptance of a fertilized ovum.

A tea of nettles and lady's mantle will help stop heavy bleeding

Vagina

Uterine tube

Bladder

Ovary

The vagina is about 3 in (8 cm) long and runs downwards and forwards to open behind the pubic bone. It sheaths the penis during sexual intercourse

The uterine cavity enlarges enormously during pregnancy to accommodate the fetus, which grows and develops there

The urethra is the opening of the bladder, and lies in front of the vagina

The neck of the womb, or cervix, is at the entrance to the uterine cavity. It remains tightly closed, except during childbirth, although the spermatozoa can pass through

The clitoris is a sensitive mass of erectile tissue like a tiny copy of the male penis

The labia are two folds of skin on the sides of these structures which hide them

Vagina

Rectum

was left to regrow. We should remember this, as some herbs are now scarce due to environmental destruction and over-picking.

THE CHINESE APPROACH

Chinese herbal treatment for menstrual disorders primarily focuses on the blood. Herbs are used to replenish, strengthen, and move the blood, and to stop bleeding. Some prescriptions help after pregnancy, which is seen as a vital time in a woman's life. Many women have complaints in later years, which begin in the postnatal period.

FEMALE REPRODUCTIVE SYSTEM DISORDERS

Premenstrual tension (PMT), painful periods, heavy bleeding, endometriosis, and menopausal discomforts are all related to the menstrual cycle. Herbal treatment for these will be discussed as well as helpful herbs for conditions related to pregnancy, such as morning sickness, birth, and breastfeeding. Treatment for low fertility and low sex drive will also be given.

HERBAL TREATMENT

Many of the disorders or problems related to the reproductive system are caused by hormone imbalances. There are several herbs which help to regulate hormone activity, such as ginseng, chaste berry (Vitex agnus castus), black cohosh, and wild yam. These will be used along with herbs to strengthen the uterus, nourish the blood, and clear infections. Wild yam contains progesterone which will help with symptoms of the menopause and postnatal depression.

PREMENSTRUAL TENSION (PMT)

Irritability, over-sensitivity, lack of coordination, swollen and tender breasts, and water retention are all symptoms of PMT. For some women they are extreme, and can start up to a week before their period is due. The symptoms are generally caused by an excess of the hormone estrogen in relation to progesterone. PMT can also be aggravated by stress and tension in daily life. To help reestablish a hormonal balance, take 1–2 ml (20–40 drops) of *vitex* tincture, or a tablet, before breakfast each morning for several months. For stress and tension, drink a tea of motherwort, skullcap, passion flower, or valerian during the day to help relax.

WATER RETENTION
Use teas or tinctures of dandelion, parsley, or celery seed to clear water retention, which sometimes occurs as a premenstrual syndrome. Reduce the amount of salt eaten.

A CHINESE REMEDY
The patent formula *Xiao Yao Wan* (Free and Easy Wanderer) is helpful in easing the symptoms of PMT. In Chinese medicine, the liver *qi*, or energy, helps to regulate the flow of the *qi* and blood in the body. PMT occurs when the *qi* gets "stuck," causing feelings of irritability and frustration, as well as breast tenderness, and bloating. This remedy helps to support the liver so the *qi* flows freely. Take the week before your period is due.

DIET SUPPLEMENTS
Evening primrose oil, taken daily for several months, can help to alleviate PMT. Calcium, magnesium, vitamins E and B-Complex are also helpful, if taken regularly.

An herbal tea can help alleviate the symptoms of premenstrual tension and aid relaxation.

PAINFUL PERIODS

Painful periods cause discomfort that can interrupt work and sleep. For intense cramping pains at the beginning of a period, take a tea or tincture made from crampbark, black cohosh, and licorice (*see* Herbal Methods section). If there is tension, or it is difficult to sleep with the pain, add valerian and passion flower. Sometimes pain is relieved by a hot bath with relaxing oils or herbs of lavender or rosemary. If pain occurs each month, take *vitex* and/or diet supplements daily to help regulate the hormones.

A CHINESE TEA
Chinese motherwort (*yi mu cao*) helps to encourage bloodflow and regulate menstruation. It is a bitter tea, but helpful when pain is at the onset of bleeding, and eases once the blood flows. It can be prepared on its own as an infusion or with Chinese angelica (*dang gui*) as a Chinese decoction (see p.34).

HEAVY BLEEDING

Occasionally, bleeding during a period will be very heavy. Make an infusion using a mixture of lady's mantle, nettles, and raspberry leaf (*see* Herbal Methods section). The lady's mantle and nettles will help stop the bleeding, and the raspberry leaf strengthens the uterus. If the bleeding is severe or prolonged, consult a doctor for further investigations.

MOXA (CHINESE MUGWORT)
Moxa (Chinese mugwort) can be bought in a *moxa* roll, which is like a cigar. This is lit and held over the abdomen to warm and relax the area, helping to relieve spasms or cramps. Chinese mugwort can be drunk as a tea to help stop prolonged menstrual bleeding when there are feelings of cold and weakness. It can also be used to stop bleeding in threatened miscarriage.

RECOVERY FROM PERIODS
Menstruation can leave some women feeling depleted and tired, especially if the bleeding has been heavy. The Chinese patent remedy *Ba Zhen Wan* (Women's Precious Pills), can be taken to restore energy and fortify the blood. It contains the herb Chinese angelica (*dang gui*), which is a tonic for the blood.

DELAYED OR SUPPRESSED BLEEDING

The delay or absence of periods can be caused by pregnancy, which should always be checked. Some women have an irregular cycle with no other problems, which may be a natural rhythm for them. Ill-health, emotional upsets, and travel can also affect the menstrual cycle. If periods are irregular in adolescence, it may take time for a cycle to establish itself; try taking 1–2 ml (20–40 drops) of *vitex* each morning for a month. A tea or tincture of *vitex*, with other uterine tonics such as black cohosh and motherwort, taken three times a day, should help to reestablish the menstrual cycle in adult women.

COMING OFF THE PILL

When the contraceptive pill is stopped, the body takes a while to reestablish its natural cycle. Take a mixture of *vitex*, black cohosh, licorice, and motherwort in equal parts as a tea three times a day for the first two weeks after stopping the pill. Drink this twice a day for the third week, and once a day for the fourth week.

ENDOMETRIOSIS

This is a painful condition in which the uterine lining "escapes" from the uterus into other areas in the pelvis. Endometriosis fluctuates with hormonal changes, causing pain and sometimes very heavy bleeding. To help rebalance the hormones, take *vitex*. Use a combination of crampbark, lady's mantle, and nettles to help ease pain and stop heavy bleeding. There are other helpful herbs, but these should only be prescribed by a medical herbalist.

A MASSAGE OIL
Massage oils of either lavender, rosemary, or camomile on to the abdomen to relieve cramping pain. Put finely chopped pieces of the herb in vegetable oil. Place this in the sun or a warm place for two weeks. Strain the herbs from the

liquid using a fine piece of muslin. Store the oil in a dark glass container (*see* Herbal Methods).

PREGNANCY

Pregnancy is a special time. Herbal remedies have been used for centuries to help women through pregnancy and childbirth. Many herbs are safe to use and very effective; however, some herbs should be avoided (see below).

HERBS TO AVOID
Some herbs have a stimulating effect on the uterus and should be avoided during pregnancy. Here is a list of common herbs which should not be used: aloe vera, barberry, coltsfoot, comfrey, goldenseal, juniper, male fern, pennyroyal, poke root, rue, sage, tansy, thuja, and wormwood. If you have any doubts about using a herb in pregnancy, please check with a qualified herbalist.

THREATENED MISCARRIAGE

Miscarriage is often the body's natural response to a pregnancy that is not right from the start, and no amount of herbal intervention will stop this. However, if a woman is under stress, or her diet is inadequate, herbs can help to strengthen and nourish her, which may prevent a threatened miscarriage. Make a decoction using herbs to tone the uterus and

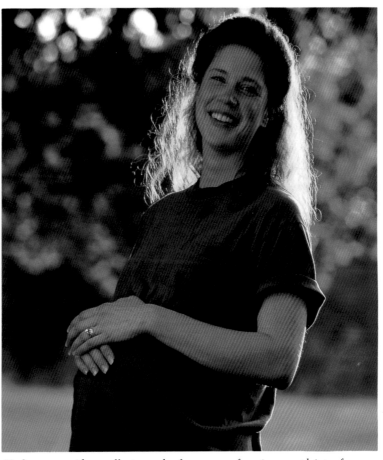

Herbs can provide an effective and safe treatment for minor complaints of pregnancy, such as morning sickness.

relax spasms. Use a mixture of false unicorn root with one-half part crampbark in 800 ml (1½ pints) water. Simmer gently for 10 minutes and drink 200 ml (8 fl oz) three times a day. Add skullcap or valerian if there is stress.

A CHINESE HERBAL REMEDY

Perilla leaf (*zi su ye*) is a warm and aromatic herb that can be taken for threatened miscarriage and/or morning sickness. Place 6 g (¼ oz) of the dried herb in 200 ml (8 fl oz) of water. Simmer for 15 minutes, then strain and drink twice a day. For morning sickness, add 4 g (⅕ oz) dried orange peel (*chen pi*) before cooking to help ease nausea.

MORNING SICKNESS

Many women experience morning sickness and nausea during the first few months of pregnancy. It is often caused by hormonal changes and low blood sugar, so its symptoms are often strongest in the morning. Drink a sweet tea of meadowsweet, camomile, or peppermint before rising out of bed. Ginger, in the form of a biscuit, capsule, or tea, may also help settle the stomach. Drink these teas throughout the day as needed. In North America raspberry leaf tea is sometimes taken for nausea in pregnancy. However, in the UK it is not used until the last three months of pregnancy (see labor, below).

Breastfeeding ensures a baby receives the right nutrients and immunity. A tea of fennel seeds will encourage the milk flow.

LABOR

During the last three months of pregnancy, drink herbal teas of raspberry leaves or squaw vine to help strengthen the uterus and prepare it for childbirth. Drink 600 ml (1 pint) of tea a day. While in labor, if contractions are weak and ineffective, drink a tea made from a mixture of raspberry leaves and black cohosh with a slice of ginger. If pains are very sharp and cramping, add crampbark. Massage the back and legs with dilute oils of lavender or camomile.

RECOVERY FROM CHILDBIRTH

For many women childbirth is not an easy process, and may leave feelings of exhaustion and depletion. A herbal remedy that is often used in China is a decoction made from Chinese angelica (*dang gui*) and astragalus (*huang qi*). The angelica revitalizes the blood and the astragalus strengthens the qi, or energy. It is especially helpful if there has been a large loss of blood or a long labor. Use 30 g (1½ oz) astragalus and 6 g (¼ oz) Chinese angelica in 800 ml (1½ pints) water. Simmer for one hour. Strain and drink warm throughout the day. Take daily until strength and vitality return.

BREASTFEEDING

Whenever possible, breastfeeding is the best way to ensure the child receives the right nutrients and immunity. To increase the flow of milk, drink a tea of fennel seed in combination with nettles, vervain, or borage. Encourage the baby to suck as much as possible, making sure that the mother is relaxed and rested.

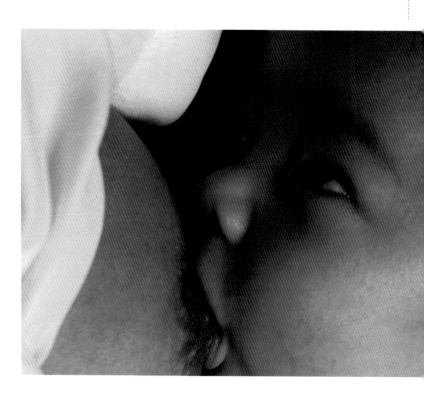

PAINFUL BREASTS

When the milkflow becomes obstructed, the breasts can become enlarged and engorged. This can be very uncomfortable and may lead to mastitis, an infection of the milk glands. It is important to keep the baby feeding, although this may be uncomfortable. Apply ice-cold compresses made from poke root tea to the breasts, or use water with a few drops of lavender, fennel, or geranium oils. Place fresh cabbage leaves or rhubarb leaves in the bra between feeds. For sore, cracked nipples, use ointments of marigold (calendula) or chickweed, or rub a drop of breastmilk into the nipple after the feed.

MASTITIS

If mastitis does set in, take a tea or tincture made from echinacea, dandelion root, yarrow, and a small amount of poke root. The echinacea and dandelion root will help to clear the infection, the yarrow will relieve any fever, and the poke root will help to clear the milk ducts. Drink this regularly three times a day until the condition clears. Apply a warm poultice of either slippery elm and marshmallow or comfrey to the breasts (*see* Herbal Methods section). Bathing the breasts in hot water and warm compresses of distilled witch hazel will also relieve discomfort.

MENOPAUSE

The menopause is a normal time of change and transition

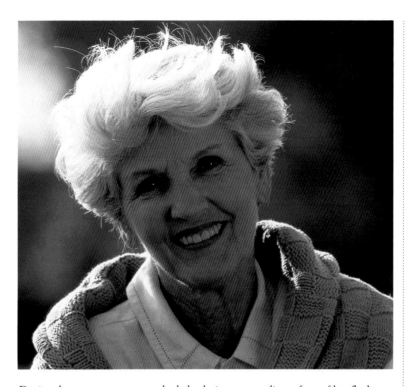

During the menopause, try an herbal solution to ease discomforts of hot flushes, depression, joint pains, and insomnia. Use the herbs over a period of time to help reestablish a hormonal balance.

in a woman's life. The first signs may be changes in the menstrual cycle, with periods becoming irregular, and hot flushes. Other discomforts may include mood swings, depression, irritability, insomnia, joint pain, low sex drive, and tiredness. For many women, emotional issues such as aging, children leaving home, and career decisions increase the pressure to reevaluate their lives. It may be difficult to separate the changes in their life from the changes in their body. A holistic approach can be supportive emotionally and physically.

HERBAL TREATMENT
A mixture of the following herbs will help the body to adapt to the changes in hormones, and to establish a new level of functioning. Use a combination of *vitex*, false unicorn root, St John's wort, angelica (*dang gui*), and motherwort for several months until discomfort is eased. Use 20 g (1 oz) of the mix-

ture with 800 ml (1½ pints) water. Prepare the angelica and false unicorn root as a decoction simmering for 30 minutes, then adding the *vitex*, St John's wort, and motherwort. Drink this throughout the day (*see* Herbal Methods section).

HOT FLUSHES
Hot flushes are a common symptom of the menopause. To relieve them, use a tea of sage and motherwort. Take vitamin E and evening primrose oil daily. Black cohosh (*see* Herbal Directory, page 114) is also useful in the treatment of symptoms of the menopause.

TIREDNESS AND DEPRESSION
Drink a tea made from St John's wort, skullcap, or vervain. Try to avoid caffeine, substituting relaxing and refreshing herbal teas, such as limeblossom, rosemary, and lemon balm. Take a good multivitamin and mineral daily.

JOINT PAINS

A Chinese herbal remedy to ease joint pains and cramping can be made from lycium fruit (*gou qi zi*) and licorice (*gan cao*). This helps to strengthen the circulation and nourish the blood. It may also help dry skin and dryness of the eyes. Prepare as a Chinese herbal decoction using 20 g (1 oz) lycium fruit and 10 g (½ oz) of licorice in 800 ml (1½ pints) of water. Simmer for 30 minutes. Strain and drink one half in the morning and one half in the evening.

LOW SEX DRIVE IN WOMEN

Low sex drive can have several causes, such as general tiredness and depression, frustration in a relationship, or hormonal imbalance. It is important to understand the cause so that treatment can be effective. Herbal treatment will help with tiredness and hormonal balance, but counseling will be more effective if there is a problem in the relationship. To help balance the hormones, take 1–2 ml (20–40 drops) of *vitex* tincture each morning. Make a Chinese herbal decoction using Chinese angelica (*dang gui*) and licorice (*gan cao*) to help overcome feelings of weakness. Drink teas of camomile, vervain, and skullcap to help relax and ease tensions. Use oils of rose, neroli, geranium, and jasmine in a herbal bath or a massage oil.

IMPOTENCE

Herbal treatment to help improve men's sex drive and libido are different. A tea of damiana and saw palmetto berries will help to boost the male hormones. Add licorice, cinnamon, and ginger to warm and strengthen the body. Use oils of frankincense and cinnamon in a bath or massage. Take regular decoctions of ginseng (*see* Herbal Methods section), for no longer than three months, to help relieve general tiredness and revitalize sexual energy. Gingko will increase the blood supply to the penis. Relaxation, visualization, and sometimes therapy are needed to deal with psychological impotence or performance anxiety.

INFERTILITY

For many couples, difficulty in conceiving can have an enormous effect on the rest of their lives. Many tests can be carried out to help find the source of the problem; medical treatment can be risky and very expensive. If there are no obvious structural problems, such as ovarian cysts or blocked fallopian tubes, it is worth trying herbal treatment because it helps to stimulate the body to heal itself. If the suggestions here do not help, try seeing a medical herbalist for a private consultation.

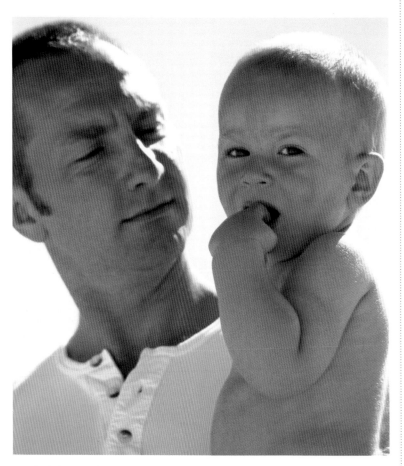

An herbal tea of damiana and saw palmetto berries will help boost male hormones, helping with problems of impotence and a low sperm count.

LOW SPERM COUNT

☙

A healthy diet, free from junk food, alcohol, cigarettes, and caffeine will help to increase the number of healthy sperm. Avoid tight clothing and hot baths. Take as a tea or a tincture a combination of damiana, saw palmetto, celery seeds, licorice, and ginger on a regular basis (*see* Herbal Methods section). Drink ginseng as a Chinese decoction or as a medicinal brandy, except in cases of high blood pressure (*see* below).

DIFFICULTY CONCEIVING

☙

These herbs help to balance a woman's hormones and nourish the blood and uterus, so they will help to encourage conception in cases where there is no known cause. Over several months, drink a tea of *vitex*, false unicorn root, roses, nettles, and marigold. Supplements of evening primrose oil, kelp, royal jelly, and vitamin B may also help.

GINSENG MEDICINAL BRANDY

☙

Take 100 g (4 oz) good-quality ginseng root and place it in a bottle of 1 liter (2 pints) brandy. Soak for two to three weeks. Drink 6 ml (approximately 1⅕ tsp) a day to help restore vitality and strengthen the body. Avoid using ginseng if there is high blood pressure, or during pregnancy.

How the male reproductive system works

The primary sex organs in the male are the two testes. They lie in the scrotum outside the body cavities where they can be kept cool, as they need to be if they are to function fully.

Each testis consists of about 200 tightly coiled tubules

The male sex cells, the spermatozoa, are produced within the tubules and emptied into the vas deferens, via the epididymis

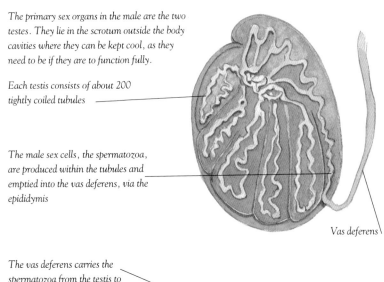

Vas deferens

The vas deferens carries the spermatozoa from the testis to the back of the bladder

Bladder

Pubis

The spermatozoa can then enter the urethra through the narrow ejaculatory ducts

Seminal vesicles

Prostate gland

The bulbo-urethral glands and the seminal vesicles add their secretions which form 90% of the volume of the semen

Drink a decoction of echinacea, couchgrass, celery seed, and horsetail for an infection of the prostate gland

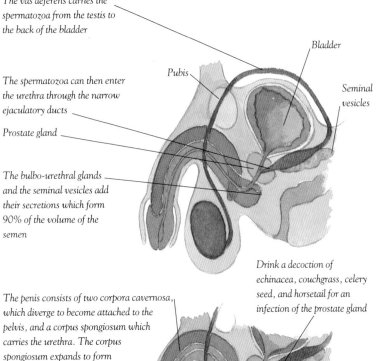

The penis consists of two corpora cavernosa, which diverge to become attached to the pelvis, and a corpus spongiosum which carries the urethra. The corpus spongiosum expands to form the glans at the tip of the penis

Rectum

Corpus spongiosum

Glans

Anus

Testis

A low sperm count will be helped with herbs such as damiana, saw palmetto, and ginseng

Scrotum

Erection of the penis is due to arterial dilatation controlled by the parasympathetic nervous system. The spongy spaces in the corpora become filled with blood at full arterial pressure.

Ejaculation expels about 3 ml of semen containing about 300 million spermatozoa into the female genital tract during sexual intercourse.

THE ENDOCRINE SYSTEM

The endocrine system, or glandular system, controls and balances the production of hormones, which have a profound effect on the state of the health of the body. The hypothalamus of the brain, and the pituitary, thyroid, and adrenal glands, the pancreas, testes, and ovaries are all parts of this system.

The processes of the endocrine system are too complex to explain in detail here. Basically, the endocrine system secretes hormones into the bloodstream, which act as chemical messengers that travel to all parts of the body. Hormone production in many cases is controlled by a negative feedback system: an over-production of one hormone will sometimes cause a decrease in another, until the balance in the body is restored. The pituitary gland plays a central role in maintaining this harmony or homeostasis.

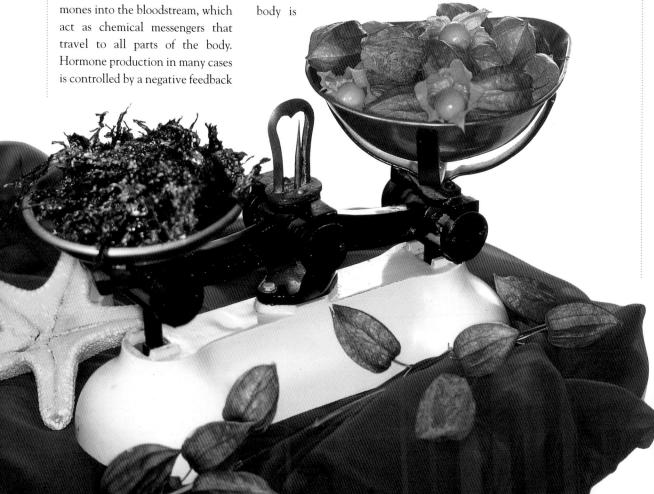

How the endocrine system works

For the widespread activities of the body, such as growth, metabolism, water/salt balance, and reproduction, which do not demand rapid changes, coordination throughout the body is affected by chemical messengers. These are the hormones produced by the ductless endocrine glands.

The thyroid gland controls the rate of metabolism. Seaweeds, such as kelp and bladderwrack, help to regulate it

Borage and ginseng help support the functions of the adrenal glands

Diabetes can be helped by a careful diet and the Chinese herb lycium fruit (gou qi zi)

PREVENTION OF DISORDERS

A healthy endocrine system can be maintained through a good diet, a relaxed and fulfilled life, and a positive mental outlook. Many disorders are brought on through stress and tension. Because of its strong link with the nervous system, it may be important to take time to relax and sort out emotional difficulties. Metabolic disorders such as diabetes or over- or under-active thyroid can be inherited or occur with no known reason, but will be helped by a healthy, well-balanced diet.

AILMENTS

In this section, treatments for diabetes, over-active thyroid, under-active thyroid, and the adrenal glands will be discussed. Suggestions for treatments for the ailments related to the testes and ovaries may be found in the section related to the reproductive system (see pp.58–65). If stress or nervous exhaustion are part of the symptom picture, consult the section on the nervous system (see pp.89–95).

INTERACTION WITH THE BODY

The effects of the endocrine system can be felt in all parts of the body. It has a strong connection with the nervous system and our emotions. For example, the adrenal glands will produce more adrenaline in dangerous situations. This then will encourage the heart to beat faster so blood gets to the muscles to encourage their quick movements, along with feelings of fear and excitement. The sexual hormones in the testes and ovaries are responsible for the reproductive process, and have a strong connection to romantic feelings. The hormones secreted by the thyroid and pancreas affect our metabolism and

blood sugar levels. The functioning of these glands will also alter our moods and state of mind.

THE CHINESE APPROACH

According to Chinese medicine, the endocrine system is not related to just one system. Treatment is according to individual symptoms, as well as information obtained from the pulse and tongue. Generally, the functioning of the adrenal glands is treated specifically with herbs that support it, such as licorice (*gan cao*), or ginseng, if there are symptoms of tiredness and depletion. Various seaweeds are added to prescriptions to regulate the thyroid.

THE PANCREAS

The pancreas is a large gland that secretes the digestive enzymes to break down protein, fat, and carbohydrates. It also produces insulin and glucagon, which regulate the amount of sugar in the blood.

DIABETES MELLITUS

Diabetes occurs when the pancreas—or more specifically the islets of Langerhans, which are part of it—malfunctions and does not produce enough insulin. Blood sugar levels are higher than normal, and extra doses of insulin may need to be taken, either through a

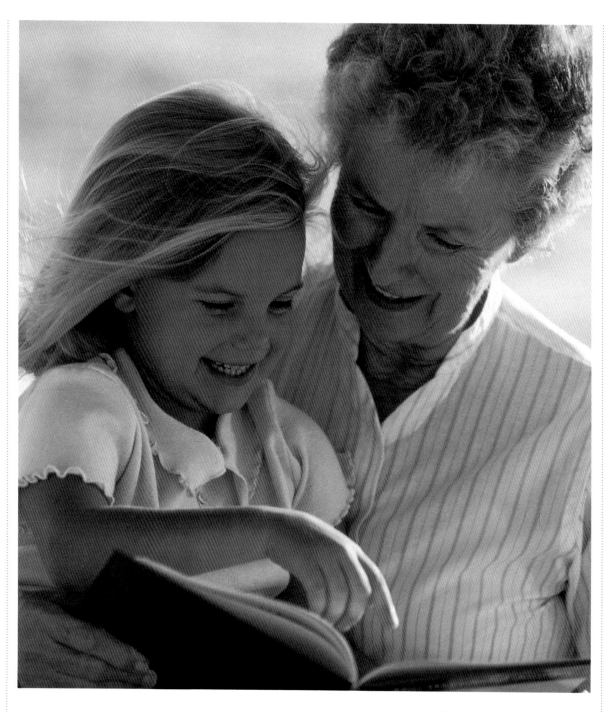

Take time to relax and enjoy life as long-term stress and strain can undermine the balancing functions of the thyroid, pancreas, and adrenal glands.

syringe or tablets, depending on the severity of the diabetes. In milder cases, usually occurring in people over 50, a diet which avoids sugars and controls carbohydrate intake may be adequate to normalize the blood sugar levels. Professional advice is needed for herbal treatment. There are records of herbs and foods such as allspice, artichoke, banana, burdock, cabbage, carrot, ginseng, nettles, oats, olives, onion, papaya, peas, spinach, sunflower, and turnip having properties that help to reduce the blood sugar level. The Chinese herb, lycium fruit (*gou qi zi*) can be eaten daily as a treatment for diabetes.

THE THYROID

The thyroid gland secretes hormones which help to regulate the metabolism of the body. They have an effect on the rate of digestion, appetite, weight gain or loss, and general feelings of anxiety, depression, and tiredness.

UNDER-ACTIVE THYROID

In this condition, the body's basic rate of activity is lowered causing symptoms of weight gain, apathy, and depression. Herbal treatment consists of nervine tonics and a specific herb that has an action on the thyroid, called bladderwrack, which is a type of seaweed. Combine two parts of bladderwrack with one part of damiana, nettles, and oats. Drink 200 ml (8 fl oz), three times a day. Take plenty of gentle exercise, such as yoga or *t'ai chi*, to help stimulate and keep energy moving.

OVER-ACTIVE THYROID

This is the opposite of the condition above, where there is an over-production of thyroid hormones. Symptoms include over-activity, with restlessness, anxiety, tension, and weight loss. Take a combination of nervine relaxants with kelp for an over-active thyroid. A helpful combination would be two parts of kelp to one part each of nettles, valerian, and yarrow.

THE ADRENAL GLANDS

The adrenal glands are located just above the kidneys and secrete the hormone adrenaline. In stressful situations, adrenaline is released into the bloodstream to prepare the body for fight-or-flight by increasing the heart rate, raising blood pressure, and stimulating breathing. Long-term stressful situations will exhaust the body and deplete the adrenal glands.

HERBAL TREATMENT

There are several herbs which support the function of the adrenal glands. Borage and ginseng are beneficial in long-term stressful situations. Take them as teas or tinctures to help build up the adrenal glands and revitalize the body. Licorice or Chinese licorice (*gan cao*) also is used as a tonic for the adrenal glands, and is especially helpful to recover from the side-effects of steroid drugs.

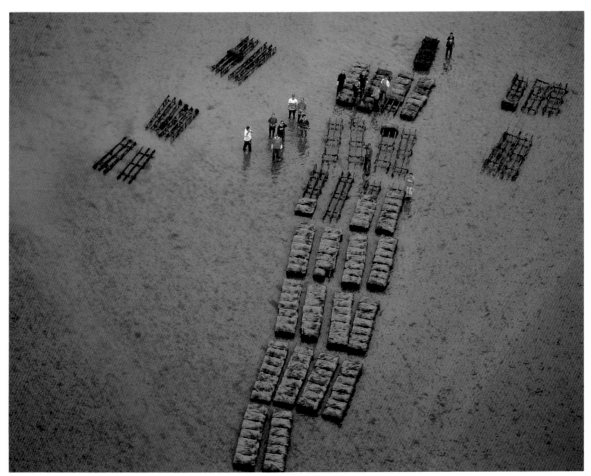

Kelp and bladderwrack are two types of seaweed which help to regulate the function of the thyroid gland. Take these in combination with other herbs.

THE SKIN

The skin is the body's largest organ, completely encasing the other organs and tissues. Its many functions include protection, excretion, and sensory perception. Ailments are rarely symptomatic of the skin itself; more often they are signs of complex processes involving aspects of the whole body.

There are two layers of the skin, the epidermis and the dermis. The epidermis is the outer layer and has four or five layers, with more on the soles of the feet and palms of the hands. The dermis is the innermost layer containing the blood vessels, nerves, glands, and hair follicles. There are two types of glands in the skin. The sebaceous glands secrete an oil to keep the skin soft and supple. The sudoriferous, or sweat, glands pass through the dermis and open as a pore through which salts, water, and acids are excreted as perspiration.

INTERACTION WITH THE BODY

The skin is responsible for excreting about one-quarter of the body's wastes. Any problem with the skin puts a strain on the other three major organs involved in eliminating wastes, the kidneys, lungs, and bowels. Any dysfunction with these organs will also have an effect on the skin. The skin helps to regulate body temperature through perspiration, which acts as a cooling process. It protects the more vital organs from extremes in temperature, harmful sun rays, and invasive micro-organisms.

THE CHINESE APPROACH

Chinese medicine sees the skin as the outer lung, which helps to explain the high correlation between asthma and eczema in many children. Chinese herbs are particularly good for skin conditions. Many herbs used to treat the skin are used to help other organs to function more efficiently. Often the diagnosis is based on the appearance of the skin, as well as other, traditional, techniques. A bright-red rash that bleeds easily will be due to too much heat; a weeping skin will be caused by

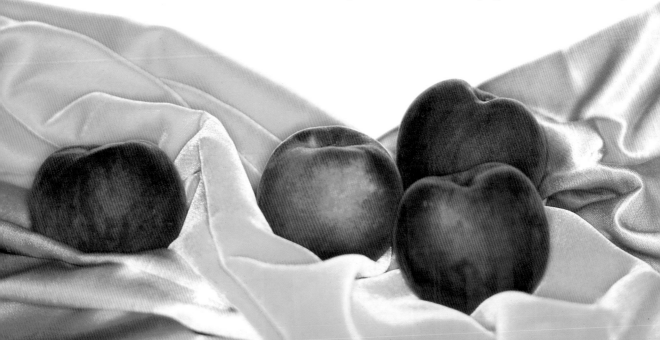

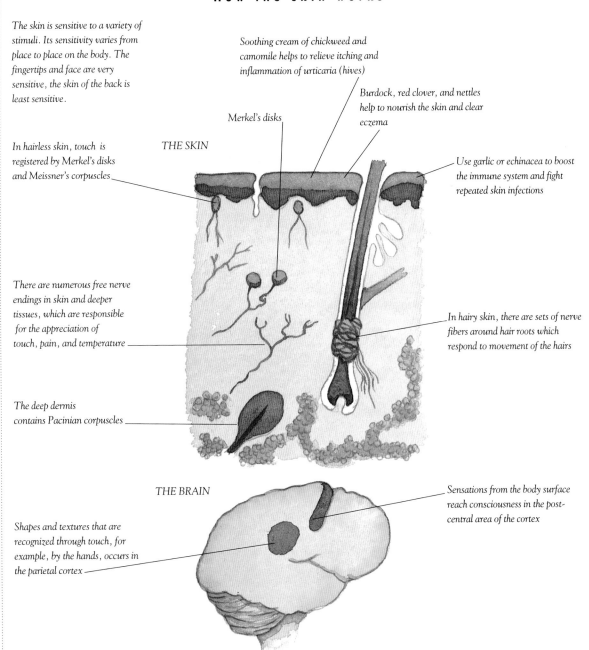

The skin is sensitive to a variety of stimuli. Its sensitivity varies from place to place on the body. The fingertips and face are very sensitive, the skin of the back is least sensitive.

Soothing cream of chickweed and camomile helps to relieve itching and inflammation of urticaria (hives)

Burdock, red clover, and nettles help to nourish the skin and clear eczema

Merkel's disks

THE SKIN

In hairless skin, touch is registered by Merkel's disks and Meissner's corpuscles

Use garlic or echinacea to boost the immune system and fight repeated skin infections

There are numerous free nerve endings in skin and deeper tissues, which are responsible for the appreciation of touch, pain, and temperature

In hairy skin, there are sets of nerve fibers around hair roots which respond to movement of the hairs

The deep dermis contains Pacinian corpuscles

THE BRAIN

Sensations from the body surface reach consciousness in the post-central area of the cortex

Shapes and textures that are recognized through touch, for example, by the hands, occurs in the parietal cortex

excessive dampness; and dry, brittle skin will indicate a lack of moisture. The herbs used will heal the whole body by clearing or tonifying, depending on the needs of the individual. Changes in the skin condition as it heals will need different herbal prescriptions. It is advisable therefore to have an individual consultation with a Chinese herbalist.

PREVENTION OF
SKIN DISEASE
There are many different types of skin disease, which means there are many causes. It is difficult to generalize because what may work for one person does not necessarily work for others. Some skin conditions indicate an inherited tendency, such as eczema and psoriasis. Others, such as acne, may

be worse at certain times in a person's life. Each skin condition will need specific advice for treatment and prevention. A good diet, containing fresh fruit and vegetables, and drinking lots of water, taking exercise, breathing fresh air, and a peaceful state of mind will all help the quality of the skin, and the quality of life itself.

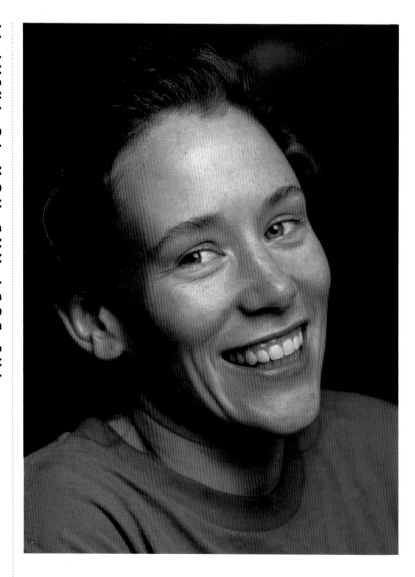

Eating a good diet and drinking lots of water will help to keep the skin clear of blemishes.

hayfever. If stress is a factor, try to deal with problems and find a more relaxing way of life.

DIETARY FACTORS

Eczema can be triggered by food allergies, particularly dairy produce, eggs, and wheat. Other foods which can cause skin reactions are tomatoes, citrus fruits, sugar, chocolate, pork, beef, peppers, and eggplant (aubergine). To find out if there is a food sensitivity, eliminate one of these foods for 10 days, then introduce it back into the diet and observe any reaction. There may be nutritional deficiencies, and supplements of evening primrose oil, vitamins A, B, C, and E, and the minerals zinc, magnesium, calcium, and iron may help.

HERBAL TREATMENTS

A hot herbal tea of echinacea and yarrow will help cleanse the blood and support the immune system. Add borage or licorice to support the adrenal glands, especially if steroid creams have been used or are being reduced. Burdock, red clover, and nettles will help to cleanse and nourish the skin. Make a decoction of several herbs and drink 600 ml (1 pint) a day. Externally, use a few drops of camomile or lemon balm oil to soothe dry skin. Aloe vera gel or comfrey ointment are also helpful. If the eczema is infected, try a bath with lavender oil, sea salt, or cider vinegar. Use a compress of marigold, burdock, or yellow dock on the infected area.

AILMENTS

Skin problems vary enormously, from those that are chronic, such as eczema and psoriasis, to those which might be a quick allergic reaction, such as a rash or urticaria (hives). Bacterial, viral, and fungal infections may cause acne, boils, warts, herpes, and athlete's foot. These conditions are all covered along with external skin problems such as bruises, burns, and wounds.

ECZEMA

Eczema is an itchy skin condition which has various forms and stages. It can appear as a red, itchy rash or weepy blisters, which then change to dry, cracked skin as they heal. Longstanding eczma can appear as dry, scaly, hard, thickened skin. If the skin is broken by scratching, it can become infected and create further inflammation. Eczema may have many causes, and it is important to find out what may help and what may aggravate it. Try to wear cotton clothing. Use a pure soap and laundry detergent for sensitive skins. Water, especially if it is very chlorinated, can dry the skin, so use oil in the bath and moisturizing creams afterward. Avoid scratching by wearing light cotton clothing that covers itchy areas. Eczema may be aggravated by animals or

PSORIASIS

Psoriasis is one of the most common skin conditions to affect white people, although it does occur in other races. It is distressing because of its appearance: red areas, often raised and clearly marked, produce excess epidermis, which can itch and flake off. Psoriasis often clears up with the help of sunshine and seawater. Stress, food allergies, and nutritional deficiencies can aggravate it in a similar way to eczema.

HERBAL TREATMENTS

Take herbal teas or tinctures to help relax and strengthen the nervous system. Camomile, skullcap, vervain, and lemon balm are all nervine tonics, and can be taken on a daily basis. Use motherwort or limeblossom if there is high blood pressure or palpitations. An infusion or decoction of burdock, nettles, cleavers, and yellow dock will help to cleanse and nourish the body (*see* Herbal Methods section). If the condition has not cleared up after three months, a professional herbalist should be consulted.

ACNE

Acne tends to be related to hormonal changes that occur during adolescence or in the menopause. Diet can also play an important role. Try to avoid fatty foods, dairy produce, chocolate, alcohol, sweets, tea, and coffee; eat plenty of fresh fruits and vegetables. Take a herbal tea made from a combination of dandelion root, burdock, cleavers, and echinacea to cleanse the blood. To help regulate hormonal imbalance, women can take chaste berry (*Vitex*

agnus castus) daily. Steam your face for five to ten minutes to clean the pores with hot infusions of lavender, camomile, or thyme. Rinse your face with rosewater, honeywater, or a dilute infusion of marigold tea to tone and close the pores. Do this every day until the skin heals (this may take several months).

URTICARIA (HIVES)

Urticaria is an allergic skin reaction which appears as a red rash. Sometimes the reaction can affect the mouth and lips, and in these cases a doctor should be called immediately because serious breathing difficulties could occur. It is important to identify the allergen, which is usually some food, perfume, an insect sting, or even strong sunlight.

AN HERBAL BATH AND COMPRESS

To relieve itching and inflammation in acute reactions, make a strong infusion of burdock or chickweed and pour it into a hot bath and have a soak or make a compress from a strong decoction of burdock root and yellow dock.

A SOOTHING CREAM

Use a combination of chickweed and camomile to make a cream to relieve itching and inflammation (*see* Herbal Methods section). The chickweed is cooling, and the camomile helps to calm and soothe the irritation of the skin.

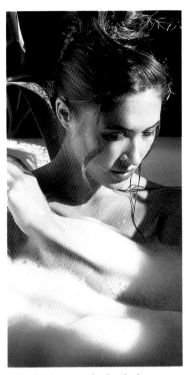

A bath of camomile, burdock, or chickweed will help to relieve acute urticaria.

ABSCESSES AND BOILS

Abscesses and boils are eruptions that are infected with pus. They occur when the skin becomes infected with the *Staphylococcus pyogenes* bacteria, often because the body is under stress or weakened. To heal these skin ailments, both internal and external treatments are needed. Use herbs to boost the immune system, such as echinacea and garlic. Drink a mixture of burdock, nettles, and poke root to help resolve the infection. Repeated attacks of boils can indicate that the body is rundown and in need of rest and relaxation. Do contact your doctor if the boils do not come to a head in a few days, or if there is a fever.

EXTERNAL TREATMENT

There are several different types of compresses and poultices to help bring out pus and discharge. You can apply these for an hour or so, three times a day. Make a poultice of slippery elm and marshmallow leaves, and apply this as hot as possible (*see* Herbal Methods section). Burdock, comfrey, or Chinese dandelion (*pu gong ying*) can also be mashed in hot water and used in a similar manner to make a poultice to draw out the infection.

A CABBAGE-LEAF POULTICE

Take a few of the inner leaves of a white cabbage and wash them well. Remove the large ribs. Tap the leaves with a rolling pin to soften them, and place them on the infection. Hold them in place with a bandage for half an hour. Remove them and replace with new leaves.

WARTS

Warts are caused by a viral infection, and can only take root if the body is susceptible or vulnerable. Treatment needs to be internal and external. Drink teas of cleavers, poke root, and prickly ash to clear the lymphatic system and strengthen the body. Externally, apply a tincture of the herb thuja (*Thuja occidentalis*) twice a day regularly for a month. Vitamin E oil or garlic oil can also be put on the warts to help them clear up.

HERPES SIMPLEX OR COLD SORES

This is another common viral infection that usually takes hold in the body early in life. The infection remains unnoticed until the resistance in the body is lowered. Cold sores can be triggered by various factors, such as other infections, menstruation, stress, or poor diet. Treatment includes boosting the immune system by taking high doses of vitamin C (1000 mg) daily, and improving diet and lifestyle. Make a decoction of echinacea, cleavers, oats, and poke root to help clear the lymphatic system (*see* Herbal Methods section). Drink the tea twice a day for two weeks. Externally, use a lotion made from echinacea and myrrh. A commercially produced extract of *Melissa officinalis* applied topically is also helpful in the treatment of cold sores.

ATHLETE'S FOOT

This is a fungal infection which mainly affects the groin and feet. Fungal infections, however, can appear anywhere on the skin, including the scalp and under the nails. It can be highly contagious, and spreads easily in warm, moist places, such as bathrooms and swimming pools. To prevent the spread of infection, use separate cloths and towels for washing and drying. Check pets for infections, as they can be a source, and treat them as needed. Drink teas made from a combination of echinacea, nettles, dandelion root, burdock, and peppermint to boost immunity. Externally, apply oils of lavender, tea tree, or thyme. Tea tree oil can irritate the skin so it is best used in a carrier or base oil. Use tinctures of myrrh, echinacea, or goldenseal on the affected area, three times a day.

CHRONIC FUNGAL INFECTIONS

Fungal infections can be stubborn, and may need long-term treatment. They can appear as dandruff, acne, or eczema, and

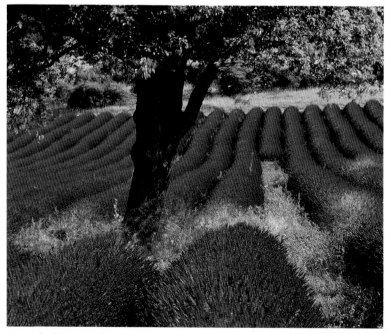

Lavender has many beneficial properties. Use lavender oil externally to fight fungal infections such as athlete's foot and as an antiseptic for skin infections.

It is important to clean a cut or wound to prevent infection. A teaspoon of St John's wort tincture in a small amount of water can be used as an antiseptic.

professional medical diagnosis may be needed. Infections can be an indication of an imbalance in the body. Eat a healthy diet, avoiding foods that contain sugar and yeast, such as breads, cakes, alcohol, and vinegar, which encourage fungal growth. Drink pao d'arco and calendula tea instead of tea and coffee to help fight fungal infections and boost immunity. Take garlic perles and a mixture of echinacea, dandelion root, and burdock tinctures to cleanse the system. Use suggested oils and tinctures to help clear external infection.

WOUNDS

There are many herbs which help with the healing of wounds, cuts, and scrapes, and also reduce scarring. Probably the most important and best known is calendula or pot marigold (*see* p.111). It is important to make sure the wound or cut is clean before using the cream to ensure there is no infection as it heals. Use a teaspoon of St John's wort tincture, or a few drops of lavender or thyme oil, in a small amount of water as an antiseptic. Other herbs which can be made into compresses are elderflower and goldenseal.

BRUISES

Apply a cold compress to a bruise to help reduce swelling and bruising. To make a compress,

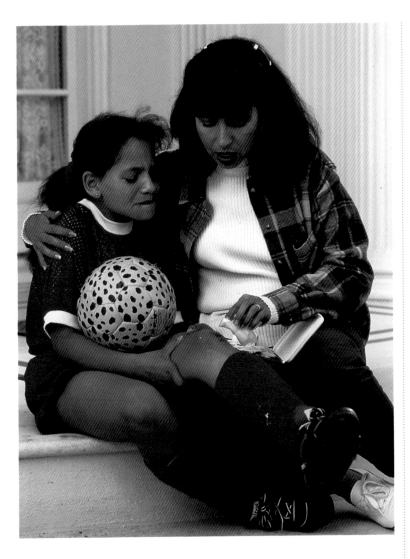

soak a clean cloth in distilled witch hazel, or in one teaspoon of arnica or calendula tincture mixed into 200 ml (8 fl oz) water. Drink a glass of water with one drop of arnica tincture to help settle the shock. Rub arnica gel, cream, or ointment into the affected area until bruising is gone. Do not use arnica or comfrey on open wounds.

ARNICA TINCTURE
Use this tincture for the treatment of bruising and sprains. Take equal amounts of fresh arnica flowers and 70 per cent alcohol, or use one part dried flowers to 10 parts alcohol. Mix together in a glass container, and seal tightly. Shake every day for two weeks, then strain the herbs through a muslin cloth. Leave this

for another two days to settle, then strain again until the liquid is clear.

BURNS

Immerse the burn into cold water immediately to help relieve the pain. Aloe vera is very effective in the treatment of burns as it helps to heal and cool the skin. Use it as a gel, or open the leaf of an aloe plant and rub this on the burn. Lavender oil or calendula ointments are also effective. Use a compress soaked in distilled witch hazel, or in an infusion of either comfrey, elderflower, or calendula, to help take away the pain and speed healing.

THE CIRCULATORY SYSTEM

This vital system transports blood to all parts of the body. The blood carries the nutrients and oxygen which feed every cell. It then carries away the waste products, which are filtered out by the lungs, kidneys, and liver.

The heart and blood vessels make up the circulatory system. The heart acts as a pump which takes in the oxygenated blood from the lungs and passes it out through the arteries into the finer network of vessels which feed the cells. The waste products are then returned through the blood in the veins back to the heart, where it is pumped to the lungs.

INTERACTION WITH THE BODY

Disease of any part of the body will affect the circulatory system. An organ which is damaged will cause strain on the circulation. An infection or a broken bone will need extra help to remove wastes and repair the tissue. If the circulatory system is weak, it will then cause strain on other parts of the body. Poor circulation will result in cold hands and feet, chilblains, cramps, and varicose veins. High and low blood pressure, arteriosclerosis, and palpitations put strain on the heart. These conditions can all be helped by herbal treatment and will be discussed in this section.

THE CHINESE MEDICINE APPROACH

In Chinese medicine, the heart is seen to be the "supreme controller." The heartbeat helps to steady and reassure the other parts of the body. It holds the *shen*, or spirit of peace, which guides and directs all that we do. Ailments and remedies related to a "disturbed *shen* of the heart" will be discussed in the section of the Nervous System.

Chinese remedies for nourishing the blood will be included here. These will be helpful with anemia and poor circulation.

PREVENTION OF CIRCULATORY DISEASE

Prevention of circulatory disease is a far better option than undergoing treatment once problems have become established. There is a greater emphasis on educating people about the importance of diet, exercise, and lifestyle. If we can take care of ourselves before an illness sets in, we will be happier and healthier. Herbal treatment can be used as part of a preventative program.

A LOW-CHOLESTEROL DIET

One of the most problematic foods for the circulatory system is saturated and unsaturated fat. There is strong evidence that an unhealthy, fatty diet can increase the amount of cholesterol in the blood, which may lead to arterial damage. Avoiding foods like sugar, butter, cream, fatty meats, hard cheeses, fried foods, and eggs can help prevent a high cholesterol level. Eating a diet of fresh fruits and vegetables, whole grains, and pulses has been shown to reduce cholesterol levels in the blood.

SMOKING

Smoking is another important factor in circulatory problems. It has a complex effect on the heart and circulation which is not fully understood. It is believed that the nicotine and carbon monoxide make the heart beat faster, while at the same time causing a thickening of the blood and increasing the chances of its clotting. Heart attacks and poor circulation are serious problems in Western society, both related to smoking.

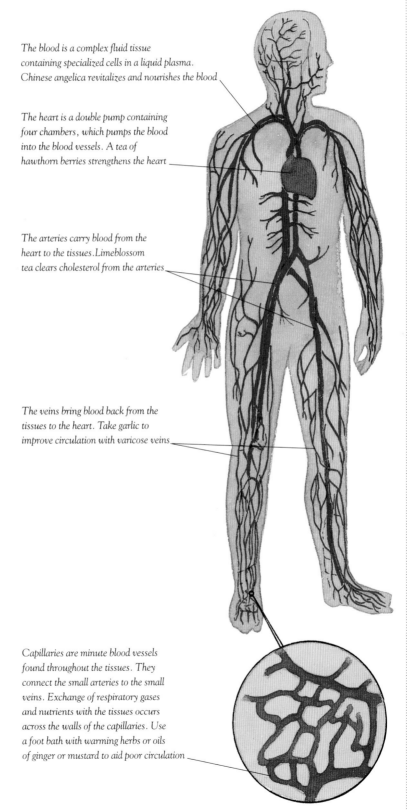

The cardiovascular system is the transport system of the body, carrying respiratory gases, foodstuffs, hormones, and other material to and from the body tissues.

The blood is a complex fluid tissue containing specialized cells in a liquid plasma. Chinese angelica revitalizes and nourishes the blood

The heart is a double pump containing four chambers, which pumps the blood into the blood vessels. A tea of hawthorn berries strengthens the heart

The arteries carry blood from the heart to the tissues. Limeblossom tea clears cholesterol from the arteries

The veins bring blood back from the tissues to the heart. Take garlic to improve circulation with varicose veins

Capillaries are minute blood vessels found throughout the tissues. They connect the small arteries to the small veins. Exchange of respiratory gases and nutrients with the tissues occurs across the walls of the capillaries. Use a foot bath with warming herbs or oils of ginger or mustard to aid poor circulation

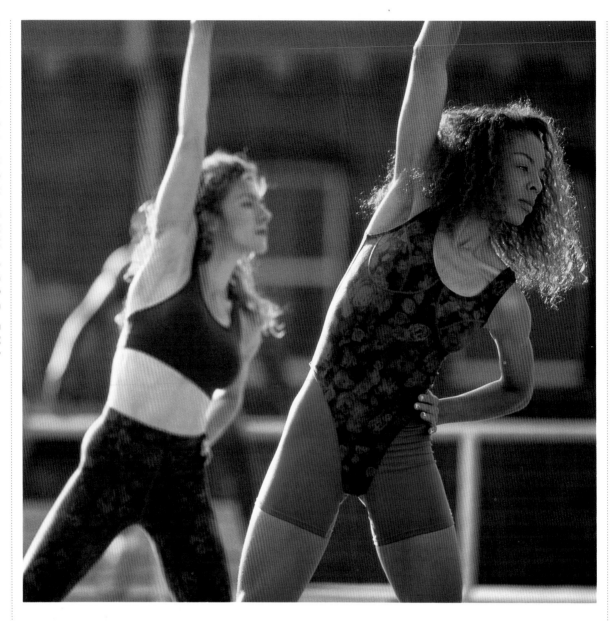

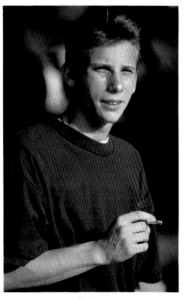

Physical exercise helps to keep us fit and well, especially as our lifestyle has become more sedentary. Smoking increases the chances of circulatory disease.

EXERCISE

Aerobic exercise, where the heart and lungs are stretched, helps to keep the circulatory system in good condition. When the heart beats faster, breathing becomes deeper and the blood is pumped into all parts of our body, enhancing its vitality and tone. Our lifestyle has become more sedentary; we walk less and drive more, and our work is less physically demanding. We need to make a conscious effort to exercise and keep fit.

COPING WITH STRESS

Stress is another factor which can aggravate health problems related to the cardiovascular system. Symptoms include palpitations, chest pains and constriction, and cramping. While there are many theories on whether stress is good or bad, what seems to be important is how we cope with stress. Herbal remedies will help to ease and alleviate symptoms of stress, but it is

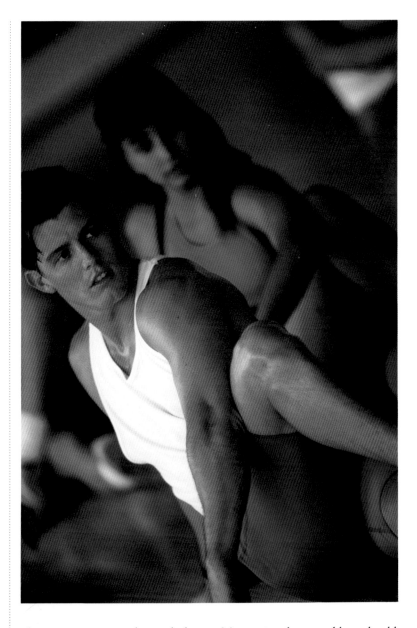

Aerobic exercise causes the heart to beat faster and breathing to become deeper, so that oxygen is circulated efficiently around the body.

tachycardia would indicate that the palpitations are due to stress and anxiety. These can be unsettling, and herbal treatment will help to relax and steady the heartbeat. Just as important, it is necessary to give up nicotine and caffeine, because they stimulate and excite the heart. Do not use hawthorn if you are receiving prescription heart medicines without advice from a herbal practitioner.

HERBAL TREATMENT
An infusion using two parts of motherwort added to one part valerian will make a relaxing and soothing tea (*see* Herbal Methods section). If there are high levels of stress and anxiety, any of the relaxing herbs, such as skullcap, passion flower, camomile, or limeblossom, may be helpful. Make an infusion using one or more of these herbs alone, or in a combination. Drink this three times a day, or as often as needed. If there is any weakness of the heart, arteriosclerosis, or heightened blood pressure, use hawthorn berries as well. They are an excellent heart tonic, and help to normalize the heart function.

also necessary to understand the causes, and deal with these.

AILMENTS
Herbal medicine has much to offer in terms of preventing complications and easing symptoms of circulatory problems. In this section, conditions which affect the heart, such as palpitations, arteriosclerosis, and high and low blood pressure, will be discussed, as well as those which affect the periphery circulation, such as varicose veins, cold hands and feet, chilblains, and cramping. Suggestions of blood tonics for anemia will also be given.

More serious heart problems should always be treated under medical supervision.

PALPITATIONS

A fast or irregular heartbeat may have many causes, and in most cases does not place any strain on the heart. Fear, excitement, stress, and anxiety may all cause palpitations. If they occur frequently and regularly, it is important to see a professional medical practitioner. A diagnosis of nervous

ARTERIO-SCLEROSIS

Arteriosclerosis is a condition whereby the artery walls thicken and harden. Initially, deposits of calcium restrict the flow of blood to the cells. Cholesterol and fatty deposits "cling" to these deposits, which causes a degeneration of the artery walls. They can build up in the aorta, and in the arteries of the heart, and brain.

PREVENTION

Arteriosclerosis is one of the most common causes of death in the Western world. It can be aggravated by high blood pressure, a diet high in fats, lack of exercise, the excessive consumption of tea, coffee, and alcohol, and also smoking. Include foods in your diet which lower cholesterol, such as soya beans, tofu, bran and oats, lemons, garlic, leeks and onions, and seeds.

HERBAL TREATMENT

Herbal treatment includes the use of limeblossom, which guards against the deposition of cholesterol with long-term use. This can be taken as a tea three times a day over a period of time. Hawthorn berries will strengthen the heart muscle, while yarrow or dandelion root will act as a diuretic, helping

to circulate the blood through the kidneys to avoid water retention.

HIGH BLOOD PRESSURE (HYPERTENSION)

Hypertension is a common condition which needs monitoring once it becomes established. It may be caused by a wide range of physical conditions, but can also have no known cause. There are several factors which can contribute to hypertension, one being a genetic predisposition. Although this can not be altered, there are several precautions which can help to maintain healthy blood pressure.

MONITORING BLOOD PRESSURE

Our blood pressure fluctuates throughout the day, depending on what we are doing. Stress and anx-

iety may affect blood pressure. Often the process of taking the blood pressure itself will cause it to rise, especially if there is a stressful wait to have it done! It is important to monitor it over a period of time. Treatment in the early stages can be very helpful in preventing hypertension from becoming a permanent condition that needs daily medication.

RELAXATION AND EXERCISE

Emotional problems and tension cause muscular constriction, which can tighten the blood vessels and influence the heartbeat. Relaxation, yoga, and massage can help the body to release tension and increase circulation. Herbal baths or aromatherapy oils such as lavender, rose, and lemon balm can be another way of letting go of stresses and strains. Regular exercise helps the circulation, and is a good way to unwind.

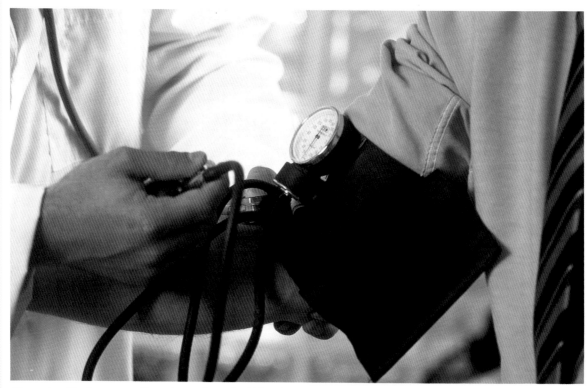

To monitor blood pressure effectively, readings should be taken over a period of time. Herbal treatment in the early stages can prevent blood pressure from becoming a condition that needs daily medication.

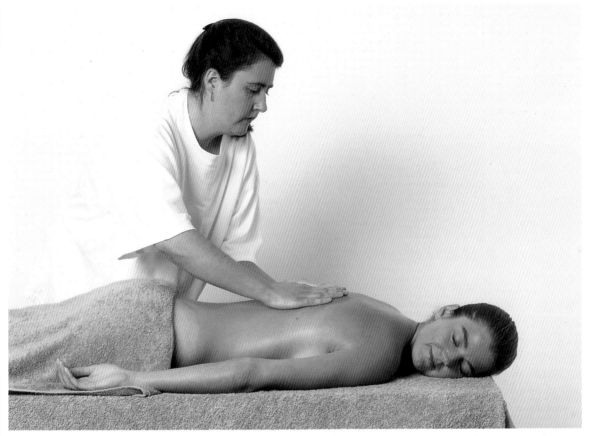

Massage, yoga, and other forms of relaxation can help the body to release tensions and increase circulation. Aromatherapy oils such as lavender, rose, and lemon balm aid this process.

THE DIET FACTOR

A diet rich in fats and carbohydrates may be a factor in high cholesterol, which in turn may cause a buildup in the arteries. Avoid these, as well as tea, coffee, alcohol, and smoking. Use olive oil, and eat plenty of fresh fruit and vegetables, nuts and seeds, whole grains, as well as raw garlic or garlic perles. Over a period of time, garlic will help reduce blood pressure and lower cholesterol levels.

HERBAL TREATMENT

Herbal treatment includes a mixture of hawthorn berries, limeflower, nettles, and motherwort. The hawthorn berries and motherwort are tonics for the heart, and help to normalize its functions. Motherwort and limeflowers are relaxants, and limeflowers are excellent for clearing any buildup

of cholesterol. Nettles are strengthening and supporting to the whole body, and help to reinvigorate the blood. Make an herbal infusion and drink 600 ml (1 pint) a day. If you are under a lot of stress, add either valerian, passion flower, or skullcap. For water retention, use diuretic herbs such as dandelion or yarrow—add them to the mixture of dried herbs. Fresh dandelion leaves can be eaten in salads.

CHINESE REMEDIES

The Chinese patent remedy *Er Ming Zuo Ci Wan*, can be used for treating hypertension. It will help to nourish the *Yin* energy, which often becomes deficient with age and overwork, and to clear symptoms of heat. These may include headache, insomnia, eye irritation, irritability, and thirst.

LOW BLOOD PRESSURE (HYPOTENSION)

This is a far less serious complaint than hypertension, however its symptoms of lethargy and tiredness can make life just as difficult. Take the herbs ginger, cayenne, or angelica as a tea or tincture (*see* Herbal Methods section). Adding ginger and cayenne to foods can warm and stimulate the circulation. In addition, drink a tea of hawthorn berries and nettles over several weeks. These will help to regulate the blood pressure and strengthen the system. Use warming oils or herbs, such as rosemary, ginger, or cinnamon in hand-and-foot baths (*see* Herbal Methods section).

VARICOSE VEINS

The enlargement and aching of veins can be caused by too much standing, too little exercise, and often is inherited. Pregnancy, constipation, and being overweight can aggravate the condition. Make sure that the feet are elevated when sitting for long periods of time to counteract the effects of gravity, and take exercise, as muscular movement helps the blood return to the heart through the veins.

HERBAL TREATMENT

Herbal medicine can help this condition when supported by exercise. A mixture of yarrow, St John's wort, limeflower, and hawthorn berries will help to improve circulation and strengthen the veins. To ease local inflammation, use a compress soaked in witch hazel, or in teas of comfrey or calendula (*see* Herbal Methods section). For severe aching, spray the area with cold water or apply crushed ice for several seconds. Massage the muscles around this area with oils of lavender, juniper, or rosemary. Take garlic to improve circulation as well as supplements of vitamins B-Complex, C, E, and zinc.

POOR CIRCULATION

Poor circulation can result in cold hands and feet. Exercise and eating green, leafy vegetables can help strengthen the blood and circulation. Use warming spices such as cinnamon, ginger, cloves, chilli, and cayenne in cooking. Add several slices of ginger root to your favorite tea. Make an infusion using equal parts of prickly ash bark or berries and hawthorn berries, and add a slice of ginger. Drink this three times a day, especially in cold weather. The prickly ash will help to stimulate the circulation, the hawthorn acts as a tonic for the circulation, and the ginger is warming. Garlic is also warming, and helps to cleanse and strengthen the blood vessels.

HAND-AND-FOOT BATHS

Make a hand-and-foot bath using warming herbs or oils such as ginger, cinnamon, mustard, or black pepper (*see* Herbal Methods section).

CHILBLAINS

Chilblains are red swellings, usually on the fingers and toes, caused by exposure to the cold. Follow the advice given for poor circulation, above. It is important to protect the hands and feet by wearing warm gloves and socks. Use rubber gloves to protect the hands during washing dishes, or if immersing them in cold water. If the chilblains are itching, soothe them with calendula ointment, or oil of lavender. If the skin is not broken, put arnica ointment, neat lemon juice, or cayenne ointment on the chilblains.

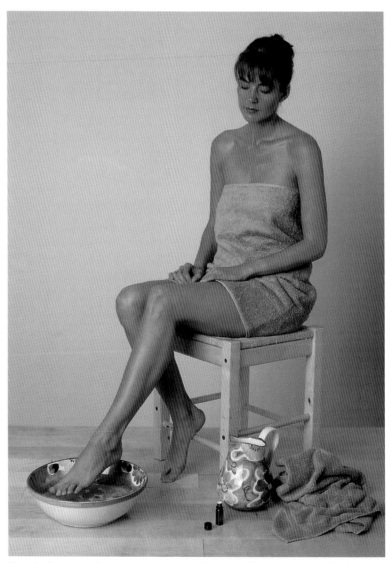

Foot baths are a relaxing way to aid circulation. Add warming oils or herbs such as cinnamon, mustard, or black pepper to help cold feet.

Cold hands and feet can be helped by the Chinese remedy Dang Gui Si Ni Tang *which contains Chinese angelica* (dang gui) *and cinnamon.*

CHINESE REMEDIES

There is an excellent Chinese herbal formula for warming the extremities. It is useful in chronic conditions in which the hands and feet are cold to the touch, and feel very cold to the person. It can also be helpful in the treatment of Raynaud's disease, and cold rheumatic and arthritic conditions. *Dang Gui Si Ni Tang* (*Dang Gui Decoction For Frigid Extremities*) warms the channels, disperses the cold, nourishes the blood, and unblocks the blood vessels. It should be used with caution during spring and summer, in warm climates, and if there are symptoms of heat, such as a red face, hot flushes, or sensations of warmth.

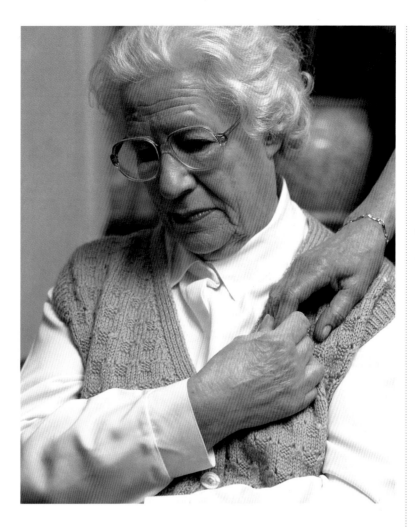

ANEMIA

In anemia there is a lack of oxygen-carrying hemoglobin in the blood. Anemia can be caused by a loss of blood, an inherited abnormality of the red blood cells, or an inability to produce red blood cells. Symptoms include tiredness, dizziness, shortness of breath, paleness, and headaches. The four main types of anemia are iron deficiency; pernicious; megaloblastic; and sickle-cell. A simple blood test will reveal if anemia is present. It is then important to find its cause, for which professional medical attention is needed.

TYPES OF ANEMIA

Anemia caused by an iron deficiency is the most common form. This can be the result of poor diet, loss of blood, illness, and infection. Pernicious anemia is due to a lack of vitamin B12. Megaloblastic anemia occurs because of a shortage of folic acid, one of the many B vitamins. Sickle-cell anemia is an inherited blood disorder which can affect some African and Middle Eastern people; this needs professional medical treatment.

THE DIET FACTOR

Dietary and herbal treatments can help revitalize the blood. Eating plenty of iron-rich foods such as dark-green, leafy vegetables, walnuts, raisins, parsley, apricots, and pumpkin seeds, and drinking red wine in moderation, will all help.

HERBAL TREATMENT

Herbal teas of chickweed, nettle, and dandelion leaves, and decoctions of burdock and yellow dock root will all replenish the blood. Drink three cups a day using one or several of the herbs in combination (*see* Herbal Methods section).

A MEDICINAL WINE

A medicinal wine to help in the treatment of amemia can be made with 200 g (8 oz) yellow dock, 4 g (2 tsp) of licorice root, 4 g (2 tsp) of juniper berries, 50 g (2 oz) dried nettles, 50 g (2 oz) chopped dried apricots, and 100 g (4 oz) of sugar added to one liter (2 pints) of red wine. Allow to soak for two weeks then strain, and put into a sterilized bottle. Drink one sherry glassful a day on an empty stomach. (See also medicinal wines in Herbal Methods section.)

THE MUSCULOSKELETAL SYSTEM

The bones and muscles give shape and form to the body. Their movement and strength varies with each individual and their age, determining physical ability throughout their lives. It is important to maintain the good health of the bones and muscles, especially as we grow older.

The adult skeleton consists of 206 bones, which are made of living tissue that is rich in blood and nerves. Bones are living things that grow and repair themselves. The muscles account for half an adult's bodyweight; their primary function is to move the skeleton. The muscles may be attached directly to the bones, or may be connected by tendons. The muscles and tendons do not act in isolation, but as part of a muscle group controlled by the nervous system.

INTERACTION WITH THE BODY

Muscles and bones form a framework which protects and holds in place the vital organs of the body. The bones are a reservoir of calcium, phosphoros, sodium, and other elements. Red and white blood cells are produced within bone marrow. The bones, muscles, and tendons maintain their strength and suppleness through exercise, and nutrients from our diet. Many of the chronic ailments affecting this system are related to these two factors.

THE CHINESE MEDICINE APPROACH

In Chinese medicine there are several energies that relate to the muscles and bones. The bones are connected with the kidney *qi*, or energy; the muscles to the spleen *qi*; the tendons to the liver and gallbladder *qi*. Ailments related to muscles, bones, and tendons may involve treatments for these different energies, but may also include herbs to nourish the blood and aid circulation. Such ailments are described as being "hot" or "cold," and cooling or warming herbs will be part of

How the musculoskeletal system works

The skeleton provides a rigid framework to support the body and maintain its shape. The main function of the skeleton is to provide a system of levers, moved by skeletal muscle, allowing the body to move.

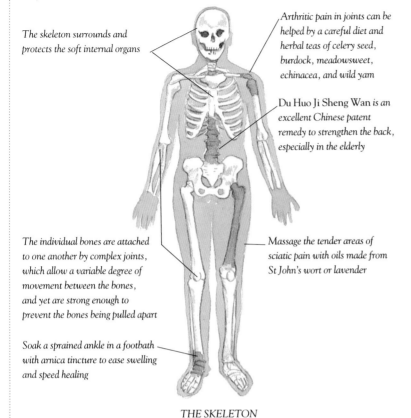

The skeleton surrounds and protects the soft internal organs

Arthritic pain in joints can be helped by a careful diet and herbal teas of celery seed, burdock, meadowsweet, echinacea, and wild yam

Du Huo Ji Sheng Wan is an excellent Chinese patent remedy to strengthen the back, especially in the elderly

The individual bones are attached to one another by complex joints, which allow a variable degree of movement between the bones, and yet are strong enough to prevent the bones being pulled apart

Massage the tender areas of sciatic pain with oils made from St John's wort or lavender

Soak a sprained ankle in a footbath with arnica tincture to ease swelling and speed healing

THE SKELETON

Skeletal muscle makes up about half the weight of the average adult. The skeletal muscles are, with a few exceptions, attached to the bone, either directly or via tendons. They move the bones at their joints when they contract. The muscles only exert their power during contraction. Several muscles are attached around a joint to permit a variety of opposing movements.

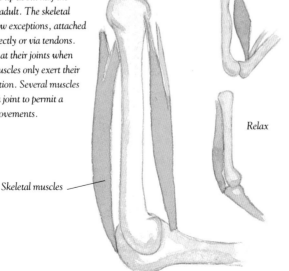

Contract

Relax

Skeletal muscles

THE ELBOW JOINT

the treatment, respectively. For example, stiff, cold arthritic joints will require the use of warming and strengthening herbs; red, swollen, hot joints will need herbs that clear heat and toxicity.

PREVENTION OF DISORDERS

The health of the musculoskeletal system is affected by the way we use it. Good posture, exercise, and a healthy diet all contribute to long-term health. The Alexander Technique and yoga can help to promote healthy posture and keep the muscles and joints supple. A great deal can be done to heal structural problems with the use of osteopathy or chiropractics, especially those resulting from accidents or injuries. Emotional stress and tension can cause rigidity of the bones and muscles; these should be dealt with before they bring about a serious condition.

AILMENTS

Rheumatism, arthritis, and gout are conditions commonly found in the elderly. Herbal treatments and diet advice will be suggested for these ailments. Treatments for backache and sciatica will be given, with some herbs to be taken as teas, and others to be used in a soothing herbal bath. Cramps and sprains are usually temporary conditions, and suggestions will be given to ease discomfort.

RHEUMATISM AND ARTHRITIS

Rheumatism and arthritis both have symptoms of painful, swollen, and stiff joints. Often the conditions are inherited, and symptoms occur as the result of the

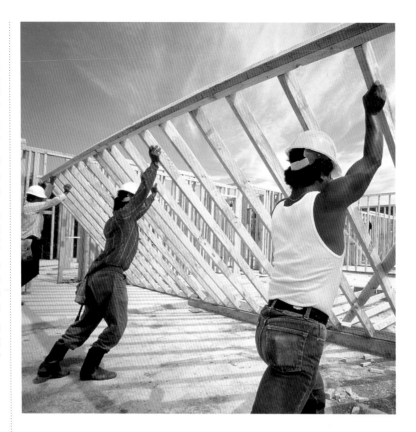

Rheumatism and arthritis may develop in later years from constant strain on one part of the body, or as a result of an accident or injury.

A CHINESE HERBAL REMEDY

A sweet-tasting Chinese herbal remedy that is useful for easing stiffness, especially in the elderly, can be made from lycium fruit (*gou qi zi*) and Chinese licorice (*gan cao*). Combine 20 g (1 oz) lycium fruit with 10 g (½ oz) licorice in a pot with 800 ml (1½ pints) water. Simmer gently for 30 minutes, then strain. Drink half in the morning, and the other half in the evening. The lycium fruit will nourish the blood, while the licorice will strengthen the *qi*, or energy.

body's inability to cope with an inappropriate diet and a stressful life. Rheumatism and arthritis can be the result of an injury or accident. Constant strain from physical work may cause an arthritic condition later on, such as the arthritic shoulder of a builder who has carried bricks on his back for many years. The weather often plays a role with the cold and damp having the worst effect.

DIETARY ADVICE

One of the causes of rheumatism and arthritis is an accumulation of toxins and waste products in the joints, which an inappropriate diet can aggravate. Generally, foods that cause an acidic reaction in the stomach should be avoided: red meats, eggs and dairy products, vinegar, refined sugar, and many spices. Foods high in oxalic acid, such as rhubarb, gooseberries, and black and red currants, should also not be eaten. In some cases, food allergies can result in arthritis and an elimination diet may help. This is best done with advice from a dietician. Herbal teas should be substituted for coffee, tea, and alcohol. Include fresh fruit and vegetables, and drink 1½ liters (3 pints) water daily. Add a teaspoon of cider vinegar to a glass of water and drink this every morning.

HERBAL TREATMENT

A tea made from a combination of celery seed, burdock, meadowsweet, and echinacea will help to clear waste from the system. Add wild yam or devil's claw to reduce pain and swelling. If there is constipation, drink aloe vera juice, or take a decoction of yellow dock and licorice (*see* Herbal Methods section). Take supplements of evening primrose oil or cod liver oil to keep joints supple. Rub joints with oils of lavender, rosemary, peppermint, and arnica.

GOUT

This is a specific joint problem caused by a buildup of uric acid in the body. It can be a very painful condition which often affects the feet. Herbal treatment includes a combination of antirheumatic herbs and diuretics to aid the process of elimination via the kidneys. Use equal amounts of burdock root, celery seed, and yarrow to make a decoction. Drink it three times a day over a period of time (*see* Herbal Methods section).

DIETARY AID

Diet is of primary importance in the treatment of gout. Avoid any foods that encourage the body's production of uric acid, such as sardines, anchovies, crab and shellfish, as well as liver, kidneys, and beans. Coffee and tea, and especially alcohol, should not be drunk. Gout may be helped by taking folic acid and vitamin C supplements.

BACKACHE

Backache can have many causes, and it should be investigated to help determine the best treatment. If it is the result of strained muscles caused by a sudden, violent movement or over use, massage the area with oils of lavender, rosemary, or St John's wort to help relieve stiffness and pain. A hot bath with a strong herbal infusion of camomile will help the muscles to relax. Use hot compresses soaked in crampbark, valerian, or ginger frequently. Make a hot salt compress by heating salt in a frying pan and wrapping it in a soft cloth. The salt will hold the heat, which will help to relax muscle spasm.

CHINESE PATENT REMEDIES

Du Huo Ji Sheng Wan is a patent remedy that is good for treating chronic backache, sciatica, arthritis, and rheumatism affecting the lower back and limbs. It contains herbs to strengthen the body, and is often used for older people. As it contains warming herbs, it should not be used with hot, swollen joints, fevers, or night sweats. It is helpful for ailments that are made worse by the cold and damp.

Another Chinese herbal remedy for weakness and pain in the lower back is *Liu Wei Di Huang Wan*. It is used for conditions with symptoms of some heat, such as restlessness, insomnia, mild night sweats, dizziness, tinnitus, high blood pressure, and burning in the soles and palms. *Du Huo Ji Sheng Wan* has warming herbs in the prescription, so is not recommended in these cases. This remedy can be used over a long period of time. (See also *moxa*, below.)

SCIATICA

Sciatica is an inflammation of the sciatic nerve, which runs from the buttock down the back of the leg into the calf. Sciatica can cause intense pain and tenderness. It is often due to a problem in the lower back, and osteopathic or chiropractic treatment is useful. Some cases of sciatica are caused by neuralgia, or nerve pain, and treatment using nerve relaxants and tonics is helpful. Drink teas of camomile, passion flower, and valerian to help soothe the inflammation and relax the muscles surrounding the nerve. Add skullcap and vervain to support the nervous system. Massage the buttock and leg with lavender and St John's wort oil to relieve the pain (*see* Herbal Methods section for a recipe for a nerve tonic oil, and *moxa*, below).

SPRAINS

Muscles, ligaments, and tendons can be pulled through accidents and injuries resulting in a sprain. Soak in a hot bath with rosemary or thyme to increase circulation to the injured area and speed healing. Arnica tincture can be used to make a hot compress or bath. Use 1 teaspoon in ½ liter (1 pint) water (*see* Herbal Methods section). Soak the sprain for 15 minutes in the solution, repeating every four hours. Arnica gel, cream, or ointment will also help but do not use if the skin is broken.

MOXA (CHINESE MUGWORT)

Moxa (Chinese mugwort) can be obtained in a stick, which is called a *moxa* roll. The dried herb is compressed and rolled in paper to make an herbal "cigar." When lit, the "cigar" is placed near the painful area, which is warmed for 10 minutes, twice a day. (To extinguish the *moxa* roll, cut off the lit end and let it drop into a bowl of water.) *Moxa* can also be used to relieve back pain and sciatica. Use acupuncture with the *moxa* to speed relief.

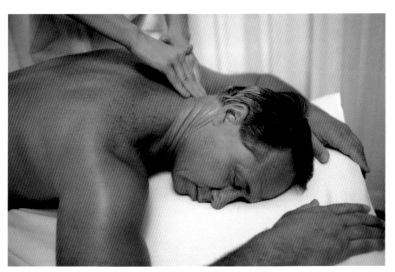

Lavender or St John's wort oil can help to ease back or neck pain, but professional help from a chiropractor or osteopath may be needed.

THE NERVOUS SYSTEM

*A holistic approach is one that recognizes the interaction of the physical
and psychological, with the nervous system as the link.
Symptoms of stress may have a physical reaction, but it is the nervous
system that helps to cope with stress.*

The nervous system helps the body to communicate and control its different parts. It is made up of the brain, the nerve cells, and the nerve fibers which run throughout the body. It coordinates our physical reactions, controls the involuntary muscles and organs such as those used in breathing, and helps us interpret and react to our environment through the senses.

THE EMOTIONAL ASPECT

In today's society there are many demands and pressures involving work and family commitments. It is the nervous system which takes the strain and helps us to cope in a way of life that is becoming ever faster and more complicated. Every aspect of our lives, from what we eat to where we live, involves greater choices and more difficult decisions than a generation ago. Taking care of ourselves means making a conscious effort to relax and enjoy our life. This is sometimes very difficult to do in our society where neuroses can seem to be the only option to its demands. Herbal treatment can be one way of helping to achieve some emotional stability in a fast-changing world.

AFFECTING THE BODY

There are a number of physical ailments which have a strong relationship to the nervous system. These include high blood pressure, coronary disease, asthma, indigestion, ulcers, skin rashes, and menstrual problems. In treating these ailments, it is useful to include herbs that relax and support the nervous system. These are discussed in other sections of the book, but it

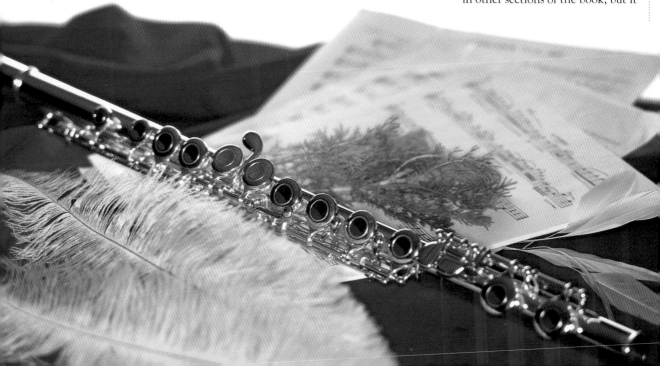

The nervous system consists of the brain, nerve cells, and nerve fibers. It conducts messages to and from the brain and around the body, and also helps maintain homeostasis, or balance, within the body.

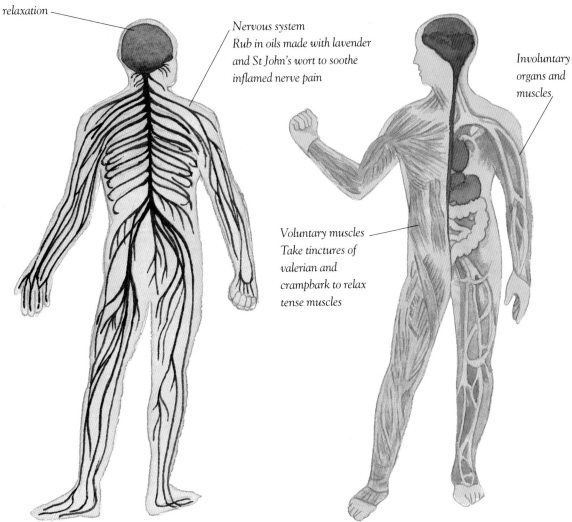

Brain
Drink teas of camomile, skullcup, and feverfew to relieve headaches and aid relaxation

Nervous system
Rub in oils made with lavender and St John's wort to soothe inflamed nerve pain

Involuntary organs and muscles

Voluntary muscles
Take tinctures of valerian and crampbark to relax tense muscles

may be useful to consider some of the herbs suggested here, especially if stress and anxiety make these conditions worse.

THE CHINESE MEDICINE APPROACH

In Chinese medicine, disorders of the nervous system are seen as the result of disturbances of *shen*, or the spirit of the heart. The heart is considered to be the "supreme controller," and a calm, steady heartbeat tells the body that all is well. Stress and anxiety, insomnia, or hyperactivity can affect the heartbeat and disturb the *shen* of the heart. According to Chinese medicine, these types of disorders can also come from a deficiency or stagnation of *qi*, or energy. For example, depression can be the result of tiredness, or may be caused by lethargy or inactivity. Many times it comes from an interaction between the two.

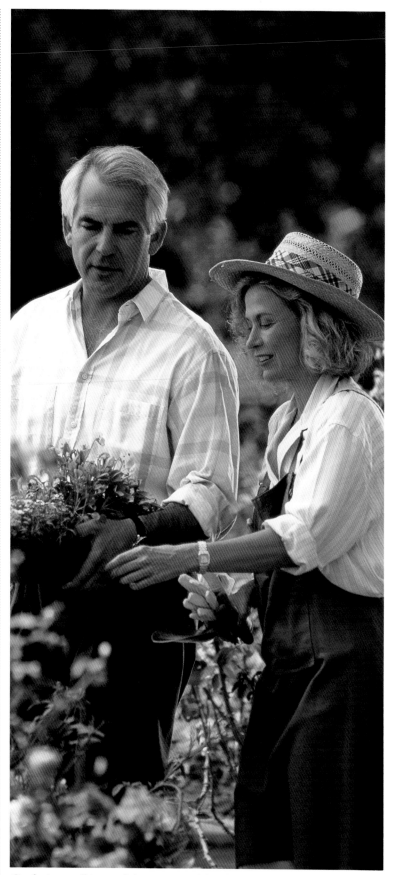

Gardening, walking, and the company of friends are all enjoyable ways to relax, exercise, breathe fresh air, and, at the same time, relieve tensions.

RELAXATION

Relaxation and meditation are two ways of relieving stress and tension. When a state of peace is felt in the body and the mind, healing can take place. Even if this is for only one hour a day, it can have a profound effect on the rest of daily life. There are many ways of relaxing, including gardening, listening to music, or taking a walk. What is important is to take time to forget about worries and cares.

BODYWORK

Exercise is another important way of helping to support the nervous system. Tense muscles restrict blood flow and breathing. Whether it is a vigorous game of squash or a gentle hour of yoga, the muscles will relax and feelings of well-being will return. Massage, aromatherapy, and other therapies which work on the body help to keep us supple and at ease.

COUNSELING

Counseling and psychotherapy can help to increase our understanding of our responses to difficult situations. Past traumas and negative patterns can hinder our ability to sort out problems in a positive way. Talking with others can bring new ideas for coping with stressful events. It is important to feel that others care and listen to us, especially in a society in which other people are becoming increasingly anonymous.

CAFFEINE AND NICOTINE

Caffeine and nicotine are both stimulants. They cause the heart to beat faster and the adrenal glands to produce more adrenaline. In a crisis the body does this naturally so there is enough energy to cope. Coffee, tea, and smoking place a strain on the body by continually creating this effect. In the long run, this can lead to tiredness and ill health. It is the body's way of saying "Stop." Herbal teas can be a delicious and healthy substitute to caffeine drinks, and a way to replenish our energy.

HERBAL REMEDIES

Herbal remedies are very effective in helping to support the nervous system through the use of nervine tonics, such as ginseng, skullcap, oats, and vervain. Nervine relaxants include camomile, crampbark, hops, hyssop, lavender, lime-blossom, motherwort, passion flower, St John's wort, skullcap, and valerian. Some of these help to relax the muscles and soothe the nerves to create a feeling of ease.

AILMENTS

Herbal treatments for each of the following disorders are discussed below: stress and anxiety, depression, insomnia, hyperactivity, headache and migraine, neuralgia, and nervous exhaustion.

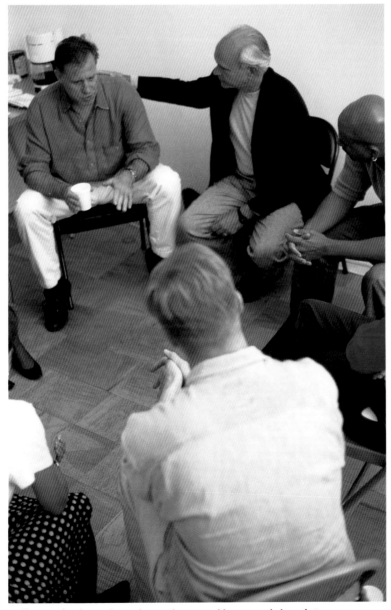

Talking with others who understand your problems may help to bring new solutions to traumatic and stressful situations.

STRESS

Stress is the body's natural reaction to any situation that places extra demands on us. It can have a positive or negative effect, depending on our response. Long-term stress, however, can put strain on the nervous system and other areas of the body which may be weak or prone to reacting to stress. Herbs can help to prevent debility, and give you the energy needed to make positive choices in stressful situations. Nerve tonics, such as skullcap and vervain, can be taken as teas, and help to strengthen the nervous system. Oats, taken daily as porridge or gruel, are an essential part of the treatment, especially if there is general debility. Vitamins C and B-Complex are also needed during stressful times.

GINSENG

Ginseng is another important nerve tonic that is used when there are other symptoms of weakness. It is classified as an adaptogen. Adaptogens help improve the body's ability to adapt to different situations, enabling it to avoid reaching a breaking-point or collapse. Take it as a Chinese decoction, tincture, medicinal wine, or powder in capsules.

ANXIETY

Anxiety can be the result of ongoing stress or a traumatic event in our lives. Sometimes it can become a habitual response, even to situations where there is no cause for worry. Using herbs to help ease feelings of anxiety reminds us of the strength that comes from feeling peaceful in our daily lives. An herbal decoction of valerian,

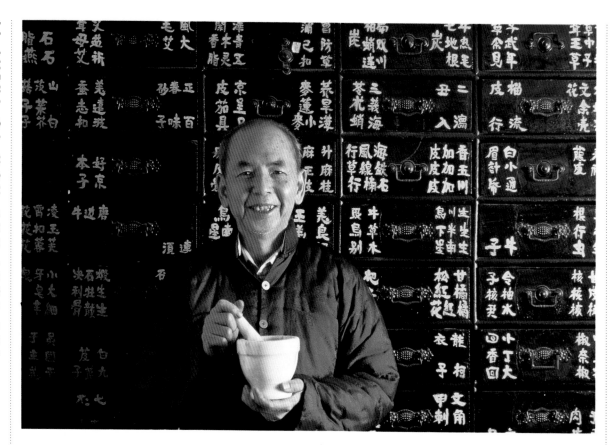

skullcap, and verbena calms anxiety and builds up the nervous system. Herbal baths in lavender, rosemary, or camomile help to ease tensions. Drink infusions of lime-blossom, camomile, passion flower, hops, hyssop, or motherwort to replace caffeine drinks such as coffee and black tea.

DEPRESSION

Depression can be the result of a long-term physical illness, general tiredness, or external difficulties. Herbal treatment can help to lift the depression and strengthen the body, creating a more positive attitude to cope with its other causes. If there is general debility with the depression, try a Chinese herbal decoction of ginseng (*see* page 34). Take wild oats, skullcap, or vervain daily as teas or tinctures to help lift the spirits and replace

nutrients. For depression following an illness, drink a tea made from rosemary, vervain, and dandelion leaves. Gingko is another herbal supplement which helps to alleviate depression, especially in the elderly. Since depression can be a serious problem, professional treatment using commercially prepared standardized extracts may be necessary. In this case, be sure to consult a health professional.

SEASONAL ADJUSTMENT DISORDER (SAD)

St John's wort will help to brighten moods, and has recently been used to treat SAD, in which depression sets in during the winter months. Add this to other herbs used for treating depression to make a medicinal tea or tincture.

In Chinese herbal medicine, ginseng has been used for over 2,000 years as a tonic to help to strengthen the nervous system.

INSOMNIA

Sleepless nights can be caused by tension, anxiety, overwork, physical pain, too much caffeine, and too little fresh air and exercise. Insomnia can create all sorts of other problems, such as chronic tiredness, lack of concentration, and depression. A good night's rest is healing for both the body and the mind.

HERBAL REMEDIES
A warm herbal bath before bed, using lavender, limeflower, camomile, or rose will ease tense muscles and calm an overactive mind. Try drinking camomile as a tea or tincture before bed (*see*

Herbal Methods section). Other herbs that can be taken as infusions are limeblossom, catnip, lemon balm, or hops. Sleep-pillows of lavender, rose petals, or hops can be tucked under your pillow at night. For persistent insomnia, try a combination of passion flower, valerian, and hops as a tincture. Take half a teaspoon in a small amount of water one hour before bedtime, and repeat again if you wake.

CHINESE REMEDIES

Chinese herbal patent formulae have several remedies useful for insomnia. *Suan Zao Ren Tang Pian* helps to treat insomnia with mental agitation, restlessness, and irritability. It calms the *shen*, the spirit of the heart. *Tian Wang Bu Xin Wan* (Heavenly King Benefit Heart Pill) also calms the *shen* and helps with insomnia that may come after a long illness or with aging. It can be used to treat insomnia and other symptoms due to a hyperactive thyroid.

Four approaches to help relieve stress, tension, and anxiety

MEDICINE
Orthodox drugs
Herbal medicine
Homeopathy
Diet
Bach Flower Remedies

PSYCHOTHERAPY
Counseling
Hypnotherapy
Psychiatry
Tender Loving Care
(TLC)

BODY WORK
Exercise
Massage
Yoga
Herbal baths
Aromatherapy
Acupuncture
Alexander Technique

SPIRITUAL HEALING
Prayer
Meditation
Music
Poetry
Gardening
Country walks
Tranquility

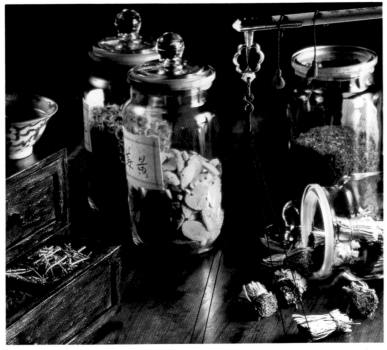

Chinese herbs are roots, bark, leaves, or berries of plants. They are combined to help balance the properties of each herb.

HYPERACTIVITY

Hyperactivity is a growing concern among parents. Lack of concentration, an inability to sit still, temper tantrums, and sleep difficulties can all be symptoms. It will vary with each child, but it often has a profound effect on both the child and the parent. A combination of good diet and herbal treatment aids this problem.

FOODS TO AVOID

Provide a diet that is as pure and natural as possible, avoiding artificial colorings and additives, which are now required by law to be listed on packaged foods. Notice if any foods spark off reactions in the child, since hyperactivity can be related to food allergies. Make sure that the child has plenty of fresh air and exercise to help let off steam.

HERBAL REMEDIES

An herbal tea of red clover should be drunk three times a day over a period of time to cleanse any toxicity from the body. Red clover is also a nervine relaxant. If stronger relaxants are needed, use oats and vervain as well. Oats can be given as porridge and the vervain as a tea or tincture. Relaxing herbal baths, using camomile or lavender, help to calm the child before bed. Try a vaporizer or aromatherapy oil burner with these herbs or essential oils to create a peaceful atmosphere (*see* Herbal Methods section).

HEADACHES

Headaches can be symptoms of an overstretched nervous system due to stress and exhaustion, but there are also other causes which need to be taken into consideration. For example, they can also be related to the menstrual cycle, allergies, high and low blood pressure, digestive problems, low blood sugar, eyestrain, poor posture, and back problems. It is important to find out the cause, especially if the headaches are chronic.

HERBAL PAIN RELIEF

Herbal treatment for pain relief includes many herbs which have a wide range of associated actions. Consult the Herbal Directory to find the herbs best suited for an individual. Suggestions include camomile, chrysanthemum (*ju hua*), feverfew, lavender, lemon balm, limeflower, passion flower, rosemary, skullcap, St John's wort, and valerian. Choose several herbs

in combination or on their own to make an infusion or decoction (*see* Herbal Methods section), and drink as needed to ease the headache. Herbal baths using lavender, rosemary, or peppermint may help lessen the pain.

TENSION HEADACHES

Rosemary, crampbark, and valerian relieve the neck and shoulder tension that sometimes accompany headache. If stress and anxiety are involved, use infusions of vervain, camomile, skullcap, and passion flower to calm and strengthen the nervous system and ease the pain. Drink as a tea when needed.

MIGRAINES

Migraines are intense headaches often accompanied with symptoms of nausea and vomiting. Visual disturbances can be early warning signs that a migraine might be about to begin.

Dizziness and light sensitivity indicate that the best treatment is to lie down and rest in a dark room.

COMMON CAUSES

Studies have shown that in most cases migraines can be aggravated by dietary factors, stress, hormonal imbalances, or structural problems. Allergic reactions to certain foods—most common of which are red meat, chocolate, hard cheeses, coffee, and red wine—can trigger migraines. Stressful situations can also be a trigger for migraines, although many sufferers cope well while the pressure is on them and find the migraine returns when they relax. Migraines related to hormonal imbalances will occur regularly throughout each month with changes in the menstrual cycle. See other sections of the book to find herbal advice to strengthen the digestion, calm and relax the nerves, and balance the hormones. Osteopathic or chiropractic treatment is necessary to check

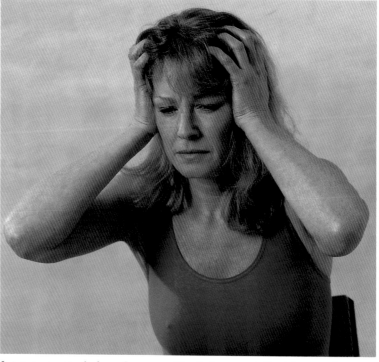

It is important to find out the cause of headaches, especially if they are chronic.

and treat any structural problems with the head, neck, and spine.

HERBAL TREATMENT
An invaluable herb for migraine treatment is feverfew, which needs to be taken daily as a tablet or tea for at least a month before its effectiveness can be seen. Passion flower, willow bark, and valerian taken as a decoction or tincture at the first sign of pain may help to prevent the migraine from becoming too severe. Continue with a small dose of herbal medicine every few hours until the headache clears. To help ease digestive symptoms such as nausea and vomiting, sip cups of either peppermint, camomile, or meadowsweet tea.

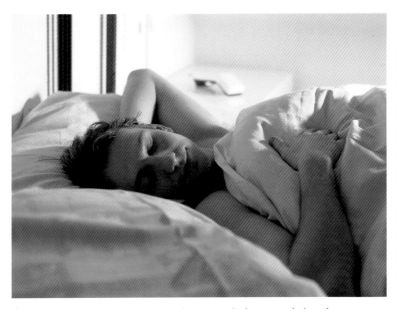

Rest is essential to relieve nervous exhaustion which can result from long-term stress and anxiety.

NEURALGIA

❦

Nerve pain, or neuralgia, can be an excruciating pain that follows the path of a nerve, or a more localized pain on the place the nerve reaches the skin. Sciatica and facial neuralgia are both common types of nerve pain. They can be caused by a structural problem that may need osteopathic or chiropractic treatment. Generally there is some debility, and this is why the nerve pain and inflammation does not go away. Include lots of green vegetables and fruit in your diet, with extra supplements of vitamin B-Complex for a while. Rest and relax to allow the body to heal itself.

HERBAL TREATMENT
Herbal treatment should include infusions, decoctions, or tinctures of ginseng, hops, passion flower, St John's wort, and valerian. Choose the herb that suits your overall complaint, and take it three times a day. Lavender and St John's wort

oil can be rubbed into the painful area, giving temporary relief from pain. If the neuralgia is associated with shingles, then take a tea or tincture of echinacea and calendula for a period of three months to cleanse and heal the body.

NERVOUS EXHAUSTION

❦

Long-term stress and anxiety, overwork, insomnia, and poor diet may lead to low vitality and nervous exhaustion. During stressful periods, vitamins and minerals are used by the body in higher concentrations. It is often more difficult to eat well during these times. Greater amounts of tea, coffee, and alcohol may be consumed, all of which further deplete the body. This may create a destructive cycle where the energy is not being replenished, and there is little left to cope with the difficult situation. If nervous exhaustion reaches an extreme level, a collapse or breakdown occurs, which then forces rest

and recovery. Rest, vitamin supplements of B-Complex and C, and herbal treatment will help aid in recovery of vitality.

WESTERN HERBAL TREATMENT
Use a tea of red clover, dandelion leaves, and burdock to help cleanse the body, especially if large amounts of coffee, tea, and alcohol have been consumed. Nettles can help to tonify and remineralize the system. Nervine tonics such as oats, vervain, and skullcap will strengthen the nervous system. Drink these herbs three times a day, and avoid coffee, alcohol, and tobacco. Add licorice root to support their effect on the adrenal glands, which are often weakened by overwork and overconsumption of caffeine.

CHINESE HERBAL TREATMENT
The Chinese herbs ginseng and astragalus will help to boost the physical energy as well as having a calming effect. Take one of them as a Chinese herbal decoction twice a day.

THE IMMUNE SYSTEM

The immune system keeps us healthy by fighting off the many organisms that attack the body, including bacteria, viruses, fungi, parasites, and allergens. It is a complex system that is well integrated into all aspects of the body, and has many levels of defense.

The body has many intricate mechanisms to fight off potentially harmful micro-organisms. Tears and saliva are antiseptic; the nose and chest have tiny hairs and sticky mucus in which to trap organisms; and the skin is coated in a protective oil. To get rid of harmful organisms, the stomach and vagina contain acids; the bladder flushes such organisms out; and the bowels contain gut flora that helps clear them. The blood contains white blood cells which attack an infection. If these natural systems fail, the lymphatic system is put into action, and antibodies are produced to fight the invading mico-organisms.

THE ROLE OF THE LYMPHATIC SYSTEM

The lymphatic system is a network of tiny vessels which carry lymph, a colorless liquid which picks up debris and micro-organisms, and lymph nodes, which are concentrations of white blood cells. The lymph nodes are situated in groups in the neck, armpits, groin, chest, and abdomen. White blood cells consume the harmful microbes and filter out debris. They also produce antibodies, which are carried throughout the body via the lymph. When the body is under attack, the lymph nodes swell and feel tender.

INTERACTION WITH THE BODY

The immune system is integrated into the body as described above. A healthy diet and good digestion are important in the production of lymph. Lymph is moved throughout the body by the contractions of the muscles. The liver is the main detoxifying organ in the body, and the debris from infections is filtered out from the blood.

THE CHINESE MEDICINE APPROACH

In Chinese medicine, the immune system is regarded as the *wei qi*, or defensive energy, that surrounds the body. It is closely related to the digestive system, and herbs that strengthen this,

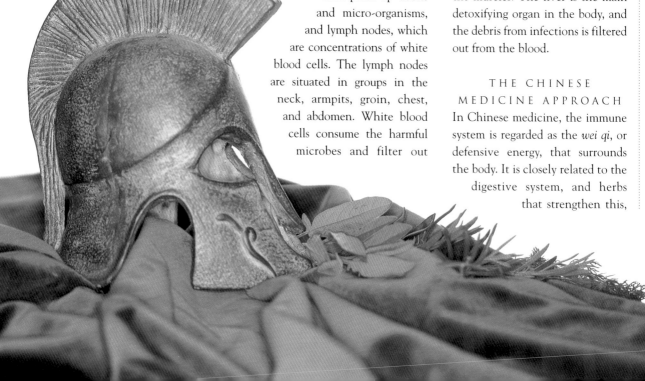

such as ginseng and astragalus (*huang qi*), help to build up this energy. If the *wei qi* is strong, infections are prevented from taking hold in the body.

BOOSTING IMMUNITY
There are several factors that impair the immune system and weaken it. Stress, a poor diet and nutritional deficiencies, environmental pollution, injury and surgery, digestive problems, and the over-use of antibiotics can all impair the immune system. A positive and relaxed state of mind will help to increase the body's ability to cope with allergies and disease. A wholefood diet high in organic fruits and vegetables, nuts, beans, and pulses, and unrefined oils will provide a good foundation for a healthy immune system. Using herbs that strengthen the immune system and help recovery from illness and injury, will enhance healthy functioning in all systems of the body.

STRENGTHENING THE
IMMUNE SYSTEM
There are many herbs that will help to boost the immune system. Garlic is one of nature's best antimicrobial products that helps to prevent infections, even for those who have become immune to antibiotics. Take one or two garlic perles morning and night. Borage has a supportive and restorative effect on the adrenal glands. It is used to help with depression and other stress-related problems, as well as to aid convalescence. Wild yam has an anti-inflammatory effect, helping to relieve symptoms of infection and allergy. It is also a tonic for the digestive tract and liver. As an alternative to antibiotics, echinacea is useful for fighting infections and cleansing the blood and lymphatic system.

How the immune system works

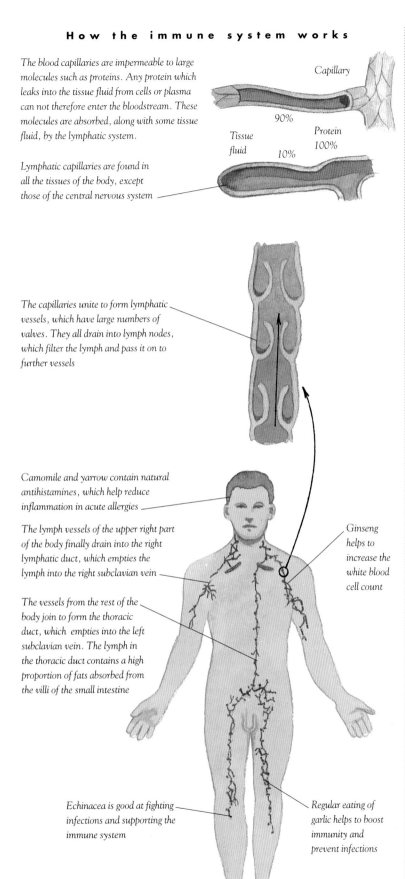

The blood capillaries are impermeable to large molecules such as proteins. Any protein which leaks into the tissue fluid from cells or plasma can not therefore enter the bloodstream. These molecules are absorbed, along with some tissue fluid, by the lymphatic system.

Capillary

90%

Tissue fluid

Protein 100%

10%

Lymphatic capillaries are found in all the tissues of the body, except those of the central nervous system

The capillaries unite to form lymphatic vessels, which have large numbers of valves. They all drain into lymph nodes, which filter the lymph and pass it on to further vessels

Camomile and yarrow contain natural antihistamines, which help reduce inflammation in acute allergies

The lymph vessels of the upper right part of the body finally drain into the right lymphatic duct, which empties the lymph into the right subclavian vein

Ginseng helps to increase the white blood cell count

The vessels from the rest of the body join to form the thoracic duct, which empties into the left subclavian vein. The lymph in the thoracic duct contains a high proportion of fats absorbed from the villi of the small intestine

Echinacea is good at fighting infections and supporting the immune system

Regular eating of garlic helps to boost immunity and prevent infections

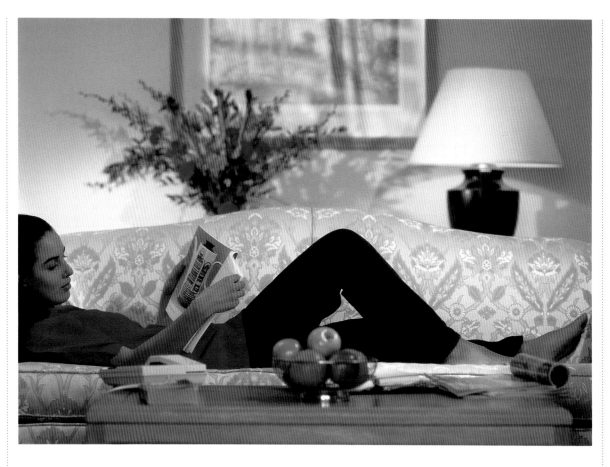

Convalescence of illness needs to include rest, a healthy diet, and herbal treatment to help boost immunity.

CHINESE HERBS

Astragalus (*huang qi*) can be used to increase energy and build resistance to disease. Chinese angelica (*dang qui*) helps to restore energy and vitality, and stimulates white blood cell and antibody formation. Licorice (*gan cao*) can be taken during recovery from illness, and helps to support the functions of the liver and adrenal glands; it also enhances the immune system by stimulating the formation of white blood cells and antibodies. Ginseng is a wonderful remedy which boosts immunity and energy and enables the body to cope with stress. It can increase the white blood cell count, and benefits the liver and spleen.

AILMENTS

In this section ailments related to a low-immune system will be discussed. Herbal and more conventional treatments for infections will be reviewed. Suggestions will be given to reduce the side-effects of antibiotics and other drugs. Ways of finding out and recognizing possible allergic substances, and treatment for allergies, will be given.

INFECTIONS

Bacterial and viral infections are the most common form of acute illnesses. Bacteria can invade the respiratory and the digestive systems, causing complaints such as throat, ear, and chest infections, and gastric upsets. Colds, influenza, and infectious diseases found in childhood are often due to viral infections. Supplements of vitamin C can be used to boost immunity. Take up to 500 mg three or four times a day. If this is more than the body needs, it will be excreted through the urine, and may cause diarrhea. Garlic will also fight both viral and bacterial infections.

ANTIBIOTICS

If there is a lot of pain or a high fever, antibiotics are valuable in fighting bacterial infections, such as those of the inner ear, throat, or chest. If the body temperature goes above 40°C (104°F), or there are symptoms of confusion, or loss of consciousness, or twitching, consult a doctor immediately. If the fever or pain lasts for more than three days without signs of improvement, professional medical advice is needed. Antibiotics can be useful for infections that are not clearing with the use of other forms of treatment, particularly when the person is showing signs of weakening from the illness.

DIETARY ADVICE

If antibiotics are prescribed, herbal and dietary treatments can help prevent side-effects and boost the immune system to avoid repeated attacks of infections. Side-effects include gastric upsets such as constipation, diarrhea, and abdominal pain and bloating. Garlic can be taken to boost the immune system, to protect the liver, and prevent gastric disturbances. Eat live yogurt or take lactobacillus tablets (acidophilus) to protect the intestinal bacteria and eliminate toxins and harmful organisms via the bowel. Drink a glass of water with a teaspoon of cider vinegar daily to help clear the digestive tract. Drink plenty of water and urinate frequently to flush the toxins through the system, and help the kidneys and bowels with elimination.

HELPFUL HERBS

The liver and the kidneys are involved in the filtering of toxins that are the result of drug therapy, including antibiotics. They are susceptible to stress from this process, and herbal treatment can be used to strengthen and support them. Chinese angelica, rosemary, and dandelion root can support the action of the liver and help it to break down toxins. Dandelion root, milk thistle, agrimony, and echinacea help to repair liver damage that may be caused by a long-term use of drugs. Celery seed will support the kidneys with the filtering and elimination of toxins. Take these herbs as teas or tinctures as needed (*see* Herbal Methods section).

ALLERGIES

An allergic reaction is caused when the immune system reacts against a substance which is not potentially infectious or harmful, but in fact may be nutritious and beneficial. The linings of mucous membranes in the digestive and respiratory tracts become inflamed and release a chemical called histamine. This can cause inflammation of the nasal passages, over-production of mucus, eye irritation, asthma, diarrhea, and urticaria (hives). Hayfever, asthma, eczema, bowel problems, migraines, and headaches can all be symptoms of allergic reactions.

FOOD ALLERGIES

The most common food allergies are to wheat, dairy produce, eggs, oranges, tomatoes, peanuts, gluten (a protein found in oats, wheat, barley, and rye), food additives, and yeast. If a food allergy is suspected, remove one of the foods completely from the diet for two weeks. Sometimes the symptom of the allergy disappears within a few days. At other times it can take much longer and become worse before it gets better. Introduce the food back into the diet in a small amount every few days until it can be tolerated. Some allergies are for life, for example, those related to strawberries, penicillin, and shellfish. It is possible to be allergic to more than one food or additive so

consult a qualified nutritionist to try out a complete food allergy elimination diet.

HERBAL TREATMENT

Combine echinacea, red clover, borage, and licorice and drink as a tea three times daily over several months to help boost the immune system. A tea of marshmallow and slippery elm before meals will soothe the digestive tract if there are symptoms of upset. Camomile or yarrow teas contain natural antihistamines, and help to reduce inflammations in acute allergies; they can be taken frequently. Nettle tea or soup also helps to calm allergic responses, and is strengthening to the body.

A CHINESE REMEDY

The patent remedy *Bu Zhong Yi Qi Wan* (Central Qi Pills) contains the Chinese herbs ginseng, astragalus (*huang qi*), angelica (*dang gui*), and licorice (*gan cao*). These herbs help to boost the immune system and strengthen the body, preventing allergic reactions from having their full effect. It is useful in the treatment of food allergies where symptoms affect the digestive system, combined with those of general signs of weakness, such as tiredness, a pale complexion, weak limbs, and shortness of breath.

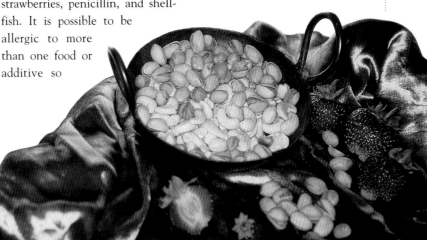

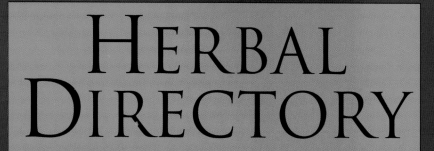

HERBAL DIRECTORY

From Achillea millefolium *to* Zingiber officinale, *this section provides information on the applications, methods of preparation, dosages and contraindications of 50 common herbs.*

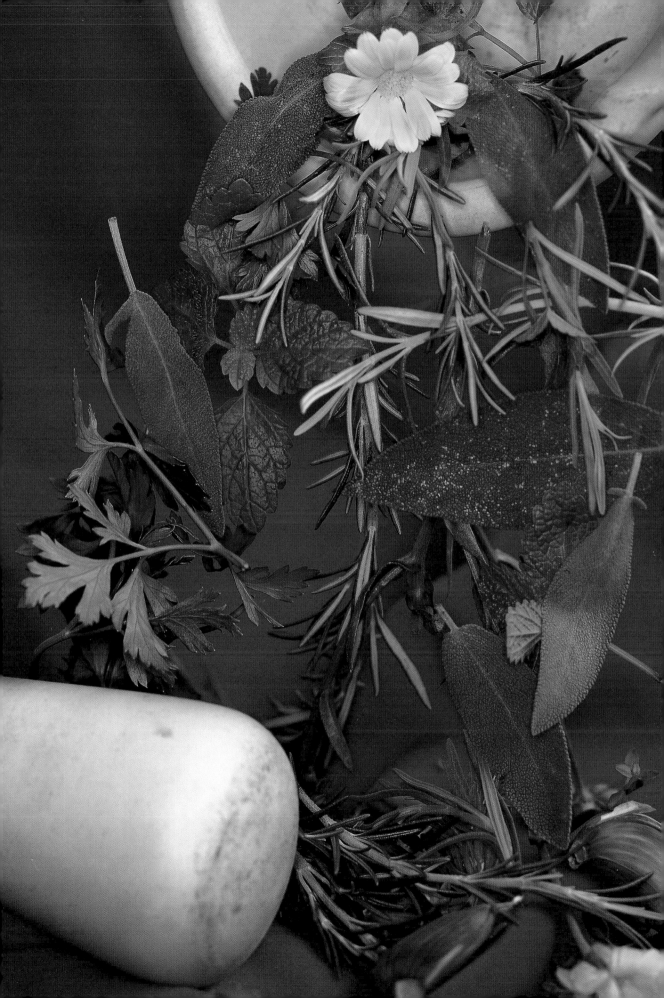

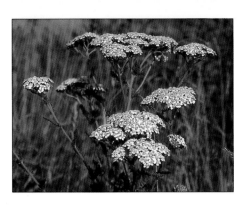

YARROW

Compositae ACHILLEA MILLEFOLIUM

This herb is a native of Europe, naturalized in North America and grown in many other countries where there is a mild climate. The herb grows to about one meter (3 ft) and can be found in various terrains. The leaves are alternate, split into many fronds, while the flowers are white or pink.

History

The name yarrow comes from the Anglo-Saxon *gearwe*, while the Latin *Achillea* denotes its reputed usage by Achilles in the Trojan war, who employed it to staunch the bleeding of wounds on the battlefield. The name *millefolium* refers to the distinctive leaves, *mille* meaning thousand, and *folium* meaning leaves. Its use to stem bleeding also gave it common names such as soldier's wound wort and knight's milfoil. Native Americans have long used this herb as a remedy. Vogel states that a report dated 1794 showed that yarrow was used on cuts by the Illinois and Miami tribes. The Ute name for yarrow designated it a wound medicine, and many tribes used it for bruises or skin problems. The Micmacs used it to promote sweating in colds and others used it for fevers.

Parts used

Herb.

Active constituents

Volatile oil, containing salicylic acid and sesquiterpene lactones; azulene, including chamazulene; flavonoids including apigenin; alkaloids, and plant acids.

How it works in the body

The apigenin has been shown to have anti-inflammatory and anti-spasmodic properties, and the azulenes and salicylic acids are also both antispasmodic. The alkaloids have a hemostatic action, which confirms its usage as a remedy to stop bleeding. Chamazulene (as in camomile) is anti-allergenic. This herb has an action in many different systems of the body. Primarily, it is probably best known for its action in the respiratory system, its diaphoretic (increases sweating) properties being used for colds and fevers. It can also be used for allergy for example, in hayfever. Its combined properties make it useful following flu or illness where there is little appetite as a tonic to promote digestion. In the cardio-vascular system its antispasmodic

and slightly diuretic action has made it valuable for lowering high blood pressure, and improving the venous circulation. In the reproductive system it is known as a menstrual regulator, which also helps to reduce heavy bleeding. Conversely, it can also bring on a period.

Applications

As a tea, yarrow can be taken with other herbs (*see* Herbal Methods, infusions: cold and flu tea p.17) 200 ml (8 fl oz) three times daily. As a tincture, take 1 ml (20 drops) three times a day.

Indications

- Colds, flu, and fever.
- Allergies such as hayfever.
- As a tonic for the digestion in convalescence.
- High blood pressure.
- Varicose veins and other vascular problems.
- To regulate periods and reduce heavy periods.

Contraindications

Do not use in pregnancy. Has in rare cases been known to cause an allergic reaction; if this occurs consult a practitioner.

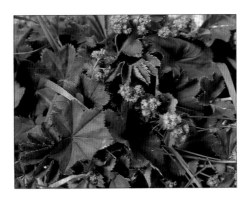

LADY'S MANTLE

Rosaceae ALCHEMILLA VULGARIS

Lady's mantle grows to around 30 cm (1 ft) high, and is a native of Britain and Europe. The lobed leaves are soft, downy, and arranged in a rosette from which the tiny yellow-green flowers rise on stalks.

History

The name lady's mantle first appeared in the *History of Plants* (1532). The name derives from its association with the Virgin Mary (note that it is lady's mantle not ladies') since the leaves are said to resemble a cape or mantle. The Latin name *Alchemilla* comes from the Arabic for alchemy, which describes the process of changing base metals into gold. In the Middle Ages it was used externally to stop bleeding from wounds and to heal sores.

Parts used

Leaves and flowers.

Active constituents

Tannins, salicylic acid.

How it works in the body

The tannins act as an astringent, helping to reduce bleeding, particu-larly in the reproductive system, thus making it a valuable treatment for excessive menstrual bleeding and in the menopause. It is an excellent tonic for the uterus. The herb's properties enable it to act as a hormonal balancer, which also means that it has the effect of normalizing an irregular cycle. The salicylic acid acts as a mild painkiller, which helps ease painful periods. The protective layer the tannins form on the tissues mean that this herb is also helpful in the digestive system where there is diarrhea.

Applications

Use the leaves as an infusion, 200 ml (8 fl oz), three times a day to help regularize the menstrual cycle and relieve heavy bleeding. In stomach upsets where there is diarrhea, take the tincture, 2 ml (40 drops), three times a day.

Indications

- Heavy menstrual or menopausal bleeding.
- To help normalize an irregular menstrual cycle.
- Cramping pains associated with a period.
- Diarrhea in digestive disorders.

Contraindications

Do not take this herb during pregnancy.

Benefits of lady's mantle

Gently astringent in gastric upsets

Useful in menopause

Eases period pains and cramps

Helps balance irregular menstrual cycle

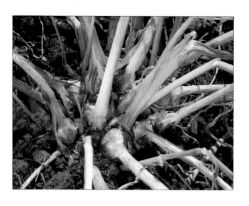

GARLIC

Liliaceae ALLIUM SATIVUM

This plant is a member of the onion family, and so well-known that it is cultivated all over the world for use in cooking as well as for its medicinal value. The leaves are long and narrow, but the part which is used, the bulb, is divided into cloves enveloped in a paper-like skin.

History

Garlic is well known through many cultures and countries. The Greeks, Romans, and Egyptians all valued its magical as well as edible properties. The name garlic is from the Anglo-Saxon, *gar* meaning spear, and *lac*, meaning plant, which refers to the shape of the leaves. In England during the First World War, garlic was used as an antiseptic to prevent sepsis of wounds. It was the main ingredient in "four thieves vinegar," used against the plague by thieves who robbed victims. Chicago derived its name from one of the names for wild garlic. The Cheyenne used one variety as a poultice for treating boils. In 18th-century Pennsylvania, it was reported that garlic and onions were given to children for croup.

Parts used

Bulb only.

Active constituents

Volatile oil, including allicin, enzymes, vitamins A, B, and C, and flavonoids.

How it works in the body

The volatile oil, which produces garlic's distinctive odor, contains allicin, which has been proved to have an antibiotic effect on *staphylococcus aureus*, among other bacterial infections affecting the body. It has also been effective against *candida albicans*. The allicin has in addition been shown to have a hypoglycemic effect, reducing blood sugar levels. Further, it has demonstrated an anti-thrombotic action, reducing blood clotting, as well as lowering blood pressure and reducing cholesterol.

Applications

As a palatable way of introducing garlic to the system, use peeled, crushed cloves of fresh garlic in vinegar, to add to salads. To benefit the immune system as a whole, add them to cooking. As a syrup, garlic can be used to counter sore throats and coughs. Take 5 ml (1 tsp) four or five times a day. It is possible to obtain garlic juice as a commercial preparation, and also tablets and capsules (perles).

Indications

- Chest infections, including bronchitic ailments.
- Coughs, colds, and flu.
- To reduce catarrh.
- To reduce cholesterol, lower blood pressure, and to prevent the clotting of blood in thrombosis.
- Digestive problems.
- In late onset diabetes, to reduce blood sugar levels.

Contraindications

Do not give raw garlic medicinally to children under 12 without the supervision of a herbal or medical practitioner. Although some people do eat garlic raw, it is advisable to only eat it with other foods as it is very strong and can cause griping pains if eaten on its own. Garlic may be taken alongside conventional antibiotics and diabetic medication, but it is warned that conventional medicines must not be discontinued without advice from a medical or herbal practitioner as this can be dangerous.

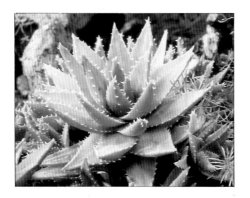

ALOE VERA

Liliaceae ALOE VERA

Aloe vera, a succulent with long, fleshy leaves, originates from Africa but is also cultivated all over the world. It is often seen as a pot plant in homes.

History

Aloe vera has been used for thousands of years. Some of its most famous users reputedly include Alexander the Great and Cleopatra. Commercially, it is added to many skin-care products.

Parts used

The leaves contain two different liquids, both of which can be used medicinally. The first is a clear gel, which is obtained by breaking the upper parts of the leaves and is used externally on the skin as a healing agent for cuts, scrapes, and burns. The second is a bitter yellow substance, "bitter aloes" which is derived from the rind of the plant. This liquid is very strong and acts as a laxative when taken internally. The "bitters" should never come into contact with the skin, and their use as a laxative should only be employed under the supervision of a practitioner.

Active constituents

Polysaccharides, the gel contains anthraquinone glycosides, known as "Aloin," and aloe-emodin, glycoproteins, saponins, and resins.

How it works in the body

The properties of aloe vera mean that it is excellent as a vulnary or wound healer, mainly due to the anthraquinones, and the gel is particularly noted for its soothing quality when used topically on the skin. Internally the gel is also useful as a healer, particularly in the digestive system. Generally, the gel is good for the immune system. The laxative effect derives from the irritant nature of the yellow sap, which in lower doses stimulates the colon producing a bowel movement. However, in larger doses it acts as a purgative, giving a much more vigorous action, which can result in griping pains. New scientific interest is in the use of aloe vera for radiation burns.

Application

The upper, fleshy part of the leaves is broken off and split apart to obtain the clear gel. This can be applied directly to the skin twice a day.

Indications

- Aloe vera can be used as a first-aid remedy, to help heal cuts, scrapes, and grazes. Also useful for mild burns.
- To soothe itchy or dry skin.
- To help with digestive tract problems such as ulcers.

Contraindications

This herb stimulates the uterus, so it should **never** be used during pregnancy or while breastfeeding. Also should be avoided if suffering from kidney disease.

Benefits of aloe vera

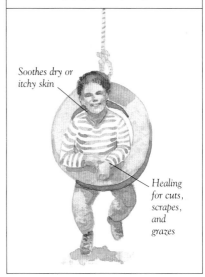

Soothes dry or itchy skin

Healing for cuts, scrapes, and grazes

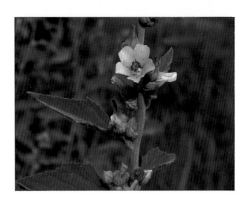

MARSHMALLOW

Malvaceae ALTHAEA OFFICINALIS

This plant is native to Europe and Britain, and is naturalized in North America. It grows to about two meters (6 ft), with pale-green, oval leaves covered in soft down, and white-pink flowers. The root is white. It is found in damp, marshy conditions, by rivers and near the seaside.

History

The name *Althaea* is from the Greek, *altho*, or to cure, and *Malvaceae* from *malake*, or soft. This plant has been used by the Romans and Egyptians as a food of great delicacy, and the roots have long been boiled and eaten as a vegetable in poorer areas. Its medicinal value has a long history, and Arabic physicians used the leaves as a poultice for inflammation. Pliny said, "Whosoever shall take a spoonful of the Mallows shall that day be free from all diseases that may come to him." The confectionery today known as marshmallow contains no trace of the plant, but the name has persisted due to the glutinous, mucilaginous quality of the main constituents. In France the flowers are one of the main ingredients of a cold remedy known as *tisane de quatre fleurs*.

Parts used

Leaves, flowers, and roots.

Active constituents

Root: mucilage 18–35 per cent, including polysaccharides, pectin, asparagine, tannins. Leaves: mucilage, flavonoids, coumarins, polyphenolic acids.

How it works in the body

The mucilage is the main ingredient which acts to soothe and protect tissues in the body. Long used for complaints of the respiratory system, marshmallow is useful where inflammation occurs in conditions of bronchitis, pleurisy, and where there is a dry cough. It is also useful in the digestive system to help heal ulcers and gastric inflammation generally occurring in irritable bowel syndrome, etc. In the urinary tract it is used to calm irritated tissues in urinary tract infections such as cystitis. In skin problems where there are ulcers or boils, it is soothing and healing, and can be used as a poultice.

Applications

For digestive disorders, respiratory complaints, and urinary tract infections, the flowers may be used as an infusion, taking 200 ml (8 fl oz) three times daily. Use also as a tincture, 2 ml (40 drops), three times daily. Prepare as a poultice for boils or ulcerations, and as a drawing paste or cream for stings, splinters, and boils. Externally, use the infusion as a wash for irritated skin.

Indications

- Respiratory complaints, bronchitic complaints, and dry coughs.
- Digestion, including irritable bowel syndrome, diverticulitis, ulcers, and excess stomach acid.
- Urinary tract infections.
- Topically as a wash for skin conditions.
- As a poultice for boils and ulcers.
- A drawing paste for stings and boils.

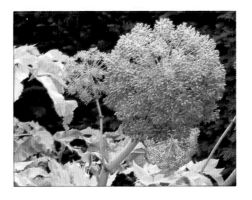

CHINESE ANGELICA

Umbelliferae ANGELICA SINENSIS *(dang gui)*

There are three main types of Angelica: European, Chinese, and American. All three are helpful for the digestion and the circulation, but there are some specific differences in how they work so they cannot be used interchangeably. The variety described here has been selected for its wide-ranging applications.

History

Chinese angelica strongly resembles its Western counterpart, but its application differs in certain respects. While also being used for the circulation, it is mainly used for women's conditions, and its use is increasingly respected.

Parts used

Roots, rhizomes, leaves, stalks, and seeds.

Active constituents

Volatile oil, coumarins, vitamin B12.

How it works in the body

Chinese angelica's constituents make it especially useful for treating women's reproductive problems. Its combined action as a circulatory and blood tonic mean it is useful in menopause for symptoms including aches, and pains, as well as helping with irregular and absent periods. Its antispasmodic actions also help with painful periods. In China it is used to nourish the blood and prevent anemia, blurred vision, tinnitus, and palpitations. Like garden angelica it is a warming, carminative herb for the digestion and has been found to help where there is long-term liver damage or infection. Chinese indications are particularly in cases of constipation. The rhizome has an antibiotic quality, and it is used in cases where there are sores and abscesses. The Chinese properties are that of sweet, acrid, bitter, and warm.

Applications

The root is added to foods in China as a tonic for the circulation. Excellent with other herbs as a wine. Take one wineglassful a day. As an infusion, take one or two cups daily. Chinese dosage is 3–15 g (⅛–¾ oz).

Indications

- Painful or irregular periods.
- Menopause, as a tonic for the reproductive system.
- As a circulatory herb for cold hands and feet.
- Improves digestion.
- Impaired liver function.

Contraindications

Do not take during pregnancy.

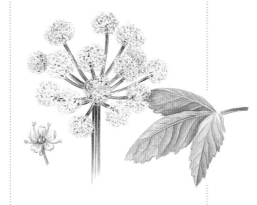

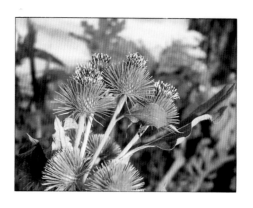

BURDOCK

Compositae ARCTIUM LAPPA (*niu bang zi*)

Chinese pharmaceutical name: *fructus arctii lappae*

Of European origin, this plant has also established itself in China and the United States. The burdock plant is from the thistle family and has large, broad leaves, and purple flowers with tiny hooks.

History

The origin of the Latin name is thought to be from the Greek *arktos*, or bear, alluding to its rough texture, and *lappa*, meaning "to take hold of." The name burdock combines burr, meaning a substance which becomes entangled, and dock, which refers to the large leaves. It forms the basis of the cleansing drink known as "dandelion and burdock." According to Vogel, an American doctor, many Native Americans used this herb—the Plains Indians used it for ceremonial purposes while the Potawatomis used the tea as a general tonic and blood purifier. In Japan, its roots are eaten for their fiber, which in tests on animals has been shown to protect the liver from the effects of food colorants.

Parts used

Roots and leaves.

Active constituents

Lignans, amino acids and poly-acetylenes in the roots. In the leaves, sesquiterpenes, bitter glycosides, arctigenin, inulin, organic acids, and oils.

How it works in the body

The plant's diuretic effect has made it a traditional remedy for gout and kidney stones. It has also been used in rheumatic conditions. Its main use is as an alterative or blood cleanser to remove waste products from the body, and it is employed to treat conditions such as psoriasis, eczema, boils, and other skin complaints. It lowers blood sugar levels, and the arctigenin has been shown to be effective against tumors. The fresh root is thought to have an antibiotic quality, probably due to the polyacetylenes. In China it is used for catarrhal conditions and when there is a fever, cough and sore throat, and in infective diseases such as mumps and the early stages of measles. Burdock also stimulates the digestion and aids the liver, and in China is a remedy for constipation. The Chinese properties are acrid, bitter, and cold.

Applications

The roots are prepared as a decoction for skin problems. A half cup is taken once a day. It is best used in its traditional way, that is, in combination with a liver herb such as dandelion. Externally use the leaves either as a poultice for boils, or as an ointment for dry skin. The tincture should only be taken for short periods, 1 ml (20 drops) twice a day for up to four weeks. As a hair rinse the decoction is thought to help with alopecia, or hair loss. The Chinese dosage is 3–9 g (⅛–½ oz).

Indications

- For its antibiotic properties in infectious illnesses to speed recovery.
- Internally for skin complaints, including eczema, psoriasis, acne, and boils.
- Externally as a poultice for boils and abscesses.
- Arthritic conditions.
- In small amounts to promote digestion and encourage the appetite.

Contraindications

Do not use in pregnancy.

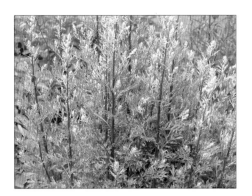

MUGWORT

Compositae ARTEMISIA VULGARIS *(moxa-ai ye)*
Chinese pharmaceutical name: *folium artemisiae argyi*

This herb of European origin grows on wasteground. It is also grown in China. The leaves are smooth green on the top and downy white underneath with deep lobes. The reddish-yellow flowers grow in spikes. It grows to about one meter (3 ft), and can be very straggly depending on soil conditions.

History

Mugwort is said to have got its common name from being used as an ingredient of beers before hops began to be used, the mug being the vessel or drinking cup. Another suggestion is that the name comes from a word for moths, as it has a reputation for keeping these insects at bay. In the Middle Ages it was believed that John the Baptist wore a girdle made from the herb, and one of its names is St John's plant; from this it probably derived the reputation of being protective of travelers, especially from evil influences. In China it is the basis of *moxa*, a substance made into sticks, which when burnt enhances the effects of acupuncture. Culpeper recommended it, " . . . for all disorders of the stomach, prevents sickness after meals and creates an appetite, but if made too strong, it disgusts the taste."

Parts used

Leaves.

Active constituents

Volatile oil, vulgarin (a sesquiterpene lactone), flavonoids, coumarin derivatives, triterpenes.

How it works in the body

Mugwort has been a traditional remedy for worms and, taken in low dosage over a period of time, can certainly help in this respect. Other functions in the digestive system include its use as a bitter, to increase appetite and promote digestion. In the reproductive system, it brings on the onset of menstruation. In Chinese herbalism the reproductive system is again the main focus for this herb. It is used to warm the womb and stop bleeding where the cycle is prolonged, and for uterine bleeding due to cold from deficiency. It is also used in threatened miscarriage, but this should be under the supervision of a qualified medical or herbal practitioner. It is also used for infertility due to a cold womb, and for menstrual pain. If used externally in the form of a *moxa* stick on specific acupuncture points, it can be used to help turn breech babies in the womb. The Chinese properties are bitter, acrid, and warm.

Applications

Use the tincture 1–2 ml (20–40 drops) twice daily; as an infusion take 100 ml (4 fl oz) twice daily. In Chinese medicine the dosage is 3–9 g (⅛–½ oz).

Indications

- Delayed or irregular periods.
- Loss of appetite, for example following illness.
- Sluggish digestion, especially where there is poor absorption.
- Externally to increase bloodflow to injured muscles, aiding the healing of strains and sprains.

Contraindications

Do not use this herb in pregnancy. **Do not** exceed the dosage. Chinese cautions indicate it should not be used in cases of heat in the blood.

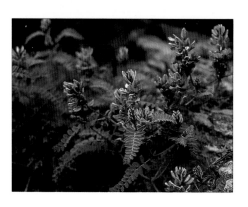

ASTRAGALUS

Leguminosae ASTRAGALUS MEMBRANACEUS (*huang qi*)

Astragalus is a native of China, and while it is not so well known in the West its use is spreading. It is found in sandy areas where there is plenty of sun. It grows to about 40 cm (16 in) high. The stems are hairy, and the leaves, up to 14 of them, grow in pairs along them.

History

Astragalus membranaceus should not be confused with the American variety *astragalus nitidus*, or milk vetch, which was reportedly used by the Cheyennes as a remedy for ivy poisoning.

Parts used

Root.

Active constituents

Asparagine, calcyosin, formononetin, astragalosides, kumatakenin, sterols.

How it works in the body

One of astragalus's main properties is that of stimulant to the immune system. American and Chinese research has confirmed its use as an energy restorative for conditions with long-term debility as a feature. It is useful in improving resistance to colds and flus and has a similar energizing effect to ginseng. It has been shown that cancer patients given astragalus are better able to withstand the side-effects of orthodox treatments, and have improved recovery times. Another of its main functions is that of a diuretic, which means that it is very active in the urinary tract, but also plays a major role in the cardiovascular system as diuretics are used to lower blood pressure. It will also help in conditions where there is water retention or oedema (swelling of the tissues due to excess water). It can be used with other herbs in cases of anemia. In the reproductive system astragalus is used where there is excessive bleeding, for example during the menstrual cycle, and also after childbirth due to *qi* (energy) and blood deficiency. In addition, it is beneficial in cases of prolapse of the uterus and other organs. It is used externally as a wound healer, especially where there is ulceration or infection leading to discharge. It can be used in the digestive system for poor appetite and digestive weakness. The Chinese properties are sweet and slightly warm.

Applications

As a decoction, one cup of astragalus may be taken twice daily. As a tincture, take 2 ml (40 drops) three times a day. The Chinese dosage is 9–30 g (½–1½ oz).

Indications

- As a diuretic to relieve water retention and reduce blood pressure.
- For colds and flu.
- When undergoing radiotherapy or chemotherapy, to reduce symptoms and enhance recovery.
- Excessive menstrual bleeding and after childbirth to reduce blood loss.
- Prolapses of the uterus and stomach.
- Ulcerative conditions and boils.
- Poor appetite and digestive weakness.

Contraindications

In Western herbalism it should not be taken internally in conditions of disorders of the skin. In Chinese herbalism this herb should not be used in skin conditions in their early stages, or where there is heat indicated by redness. It should not be used where there is food stagnation. It should be used only where there are signs of weakness.

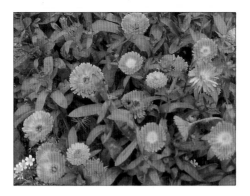

CALENDULA

Compositae CALENDULA OFFICINALIS

Commonly known as "pot marigold," this garden plant grows to about 60 cm (2 ft). It resembles a large yellow or orange daisy and has dark-green leaves. Native to Europe, it is cultivated in many other countries.

History

Its name is associated with the Roman calendar. It was later associated with the Virgin Mary, and in England with Queen Mary in the 17th century. Its use both as a culinary herb and as a medicinal plant has been very well documented.

Parts used

Petals and flowerheads.

Active constituents

Triterpenes, including calendulosides, flavonoids, volatile oil, and chlorogenic acid.

How it works in the body

One of *Calendula*'s main actions is that of an antiseptic. This makes it especially valuable externally as a wound healer, for such problems as cuts, scrapes, and wounds. Internally, it is beneficial to many skin disorders such as acne, eczema, and psoriasis. It has a well-known antifungal action, so it is helpful externally for conditions such as athlete's foot and internally for fungal-related problems such as *candida* (thrush) and diaper rash. In the cardiovascular system it is used both internally and externally for conditions such as varicose veins. In the digestive system it has helped with ulcerative conditions and also digestive complaints, and as a liver tonic. Also useful in the reproductive system, it helps relieve menstrual symptoms. It is antibacterial and antiviral.

Applications

As an infusion, take 200 ml (8 fl oz), three times daily for digestive, fungal, skin, reproductive, and cardiovascular problems. Externally, use the infusion as a wash for varicose veins and to clean cuts and scrapes. The tincture is taken internally, 2 ml (40 drops), twice a day. As a cream, use on skin complaints such as eczema and as an ointment on cuts and wounds. Also use the ointment for diaper rash and for athlete's foot. As an infused oil, apply to the skin where there are large areas of inflammation.

Indications

- Wound healer for cuts, scrapes and wounds.
- Acne, eczema, psoriasis, and other inflammatory skin complaints.
- Diaper rash, sore and cracked nipples.
- Varicose veins.
- Fungal disorders, including *candida*.
- Stomach complaints, such as ulcers and gastric inflammation.
- Regulates the menstrual cycle and lessens a heavy flow.

Benefits of calendula

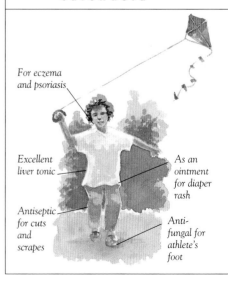

For eczema and psoriasis

Excellent liver tonic

Antiseptic for cuts and scrapes

As an ointment for diaper rash

Anti-fungal for athlete's foot

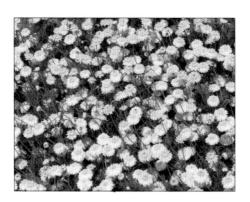

CAMOMILE

Compositae CHAMAEMELUM NOBILE CHAMOMILA RECUTITA

There are two types of camomile which are used medicinally, having broadly similar actions, Roman or garden camomile (*Chamaemelum nobile*), and German or wild camomile (*Chamomila recutita*).

History
Used by the Egyptians and Romans, camomile was dedicated to their gods. The scent is faintly like that of apples. The name derives from the Greek kamai, meaning "on the ground," and "melon," or apple. It was used in England in the Middle Ages to plant up walkways as its relaxing fragrance is released when bruised. Often it was used grown over low walls for the refreshment of the spirit. Its taste, however, is rather bitter when compared with the German camomile. Both varieties grow throughout Europe. Camomile was included in herbs taken to the New World, and in 1665 was included in a list of medicines used by an order of nuns in Quebec for their hospital pharmacy.

Parts used
Flowers and essential oil.

Active constituents
Volatile oil, principally chamazulene, flavonoids, sesquiterpene lactones, coumarins and phenolic acids.

How it works in the body
Known as the "mother of the gut," its combined properties act as a muscle relaxant in the gut, calming and dispelling nausea and indigestion, and as a sedative for the nervous system. Externally, as an emollient, it can be used as a cream or ointment for skin problems. It also has an antiallergenic quality.

Applications
As an infusion, camomile may be used by children and adults (*see* general dosages p.16). Care must be taken as the volatile oil is given off in the steam, and therefore it is important to cover the tea while it is infusing to retain the medicinal benefits. As an infusion, add to the bath to relax and calm both children and adults. As an inhalation, useful for catarrh. Externally, as a cream or ointment, use once or twice daily. Use as a poultice for slow-healing wounds, and as an eyebath to relieve tired eyes. The tincture may be taken internally up to 5 ml (1 tsp) three times a day if required, or 5 ml (1 tsp) at night to aid sleep. The essential oil should only be used externally in a base oil for massage, or in a diffuser.

Indications
- Indigestion, wind, excess acid, and stomach ulcers. Also used in nausea, especially in pregnancy, and for travel sickness, together with ginger.
- As an aid to restful sleep and to relieve stress and tension. Good for headaches.
- Respiratory complaints, such as catarrh.
- Allergic conditions such as eczema, asthma, and hayfever.
- Topically to soothe dry and itching skin.
- For tired eyes, use in an eyebath.

Contraindications
Do not use the essential oil internally or externally during pregnancy.

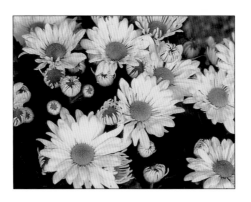

CHRYSANTHEMUM

Compositae CHRYSANTHEMUM MORIFOLIUM *(ju hua)*

Chinese pharmaceutical name: *flos chrysanthemi morifolii*

This plant grows to just over 1½ meters (5 ft) high and is known in the West as florist's chrysanthemum, as it is popularly used for flower displays. It is native to China, although it is cultivated widely in the West.

History

There are differing varieties of chrysanthemum, the white (*bai ju hua*) is used mainly as a liver herb, and is sometimes known as sweet chrysanthemum, while the yellow (*huang ju hua*) has been used to treat headaches and eye problems. It first appeared as a medicinal herb in the *Divine Husbandman's Classic of the Materia Medica* in China, AD 1.

Parts used

Flowering tops.

Active constituents

Alkaloids, volatile oil, sesquiterpene lactones, flavonoids, adenine, choline, stachydrine, chrysanthemin, and vitamin B1.

How it works in the body

Research has shown that chrysanthemum has an antibiotic principle which is affective in laboratory conditions against both *staphylococcus* and *streptococcus* bacteria, and so is a valuable remedy against infection generally in the body. In addition, the action of yellow chrysanthemum on headache and eye problems has been supported by research into high blood pressure. In one study, 46 patients with essential hypertension and/or atherosclerosis showed improvement in conditions ranging from headache and dizziness to insomnia after one week's treatment; 35 subjects had their blood pressure return to normal, and continuing improvements were shown in the remainder of the patients. This herb is also used in the respiratory system to clear fever and headaches associated with colds and flu. It has long been used as a tonic for the eyes, especially where they are red, painful, and dry, or where there is excessive watering. It is used also for spots in front of the eyes, blurry vision, or dizziness. The Chinese properties are sweet, bitter, and slightly cold.

Applications

This herb may be drunk as an infusion, 200 ml (8 fl oz), taken three times a day. The Chinese dosage is 4.5–15 g (¼–¾ oz).

Indications

- General conditions of infection.
- High blood pressure and related symptoms.
- Colds and flu accompanied by fever and headaches.
- As an eye tonic.

Contraindications

The Chinese caution recommends care when using patients with *qi* (energy) deficiencies or weakness, who have poor appetite and/or diarrhea.

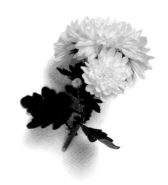

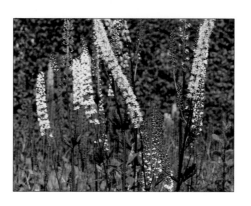

BLACK COHOSH

Ranunculaceae CIMICIFUGA RACEMOSA

There are two types of cohosh, both originating in North America. Their family and applications, however, are quite different. Here, we focus on black cohosh, a native American herb traditionally used for women's complaints. It grows in Canada, the United States, and Europe. Some related species are also used in China. It has white flowers with toothed leaves, and is noted for its black root.

History

Widely used by Native Americans, the plant was later introduced to Europe. According to Vogel, Native Americans used it for reproductive disorders, debility, to promote perspiration, and as a gargle for sore throats.

Parts used

Roots and rhizome.

Active constituents

Triterpene glycosides, isoflavones, isoferulic acid, volatile oil, and tannins.

How it works in the body

Gynecologically, in North America, it is thought that the herb balances estrogen by stabilizing it. In European herbalism it is thought to have an estrogenic action, which actively works to reduce progesterone and promote estrogen levels in the body. It is therefore used where there is a lack of estrogen and an excess of progesterone. In the musculoskeletal system it is used as an anti-inflammatory in arthritic conditions. Its sedative qualities have applications in other systems, for example, in lowering blood pressure, in reducing spasm and tension, and in the respiratory system.

Applications

This remedy is quite strong, and as such care must be taken not to exceed the stated limits. As a decoction the root should only be taken in half-cupfuls, 100 ml (4 fl oz), twice a day. The tincture may be taken 1 ml (20 drops), three times a day.

Indications

- Period pains and cramp.
- Gynecological conditions where there is a lack of estrogen or an excess of progesterone.
- High blood pressure.
- Menopausal symptoms.
- Rheumatic complaints.
- Respiratory complaints such as asthma, bronchitis, and whooping cough.

Contraindications

Do not take in pregnancy or while breastfeeding. Do not use where there is low blood pressure.

Benefits of black cohosh

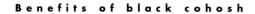

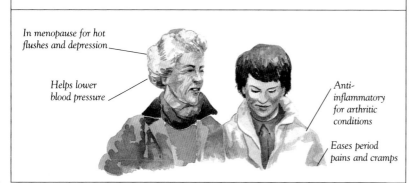

In menopause for hot flushes and depression

Helps lower blood pressure

Anti-inflammatory for arthritic conditions

Eases period pains and cramps

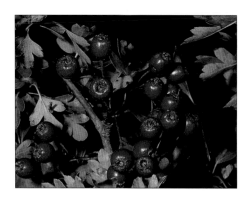

HAWTHORN

Rosaceae crataegus monogyna CRATAEGUS OXYCANTHOIDES (*shan zha*)
Chinese pharmaceutical name: *fructus crataegi*

Depending on the conditions where it exists, hawthorn grows as a bush in hedgerows and can grow to a full tree of 10 meters (30 ft) in fields. It is found in Europe, Africa, and Asia. The leaves are deeply lobed, and the flowers are white in the summer, giving way to bright red berries in the fall. The berries contain either one seed (monogyna) or two seeds (oxycanthoides).

History

The tree is regarded as sacred in the Christian tradition, as it is said to have formed the crown of thorns worn by Christ. Henry VII used it as a symbol of power after finding a badge from Richard III's helmet hanging on it after his defeat. The name *Crataegus oxycanthoides* comes from the Greek, *kratos*, being hard, *oxus* meaning sharp, and *akantha*, meaning thorn. The common name, hawthorn, comes from "haw," meaning a hedge. It is said that the mealy fruit was added to bread in England during the First World War, and that this helped to bring down the blood pressure of the population as a whole. Traditionally, hawthorn has been known to herbalists as the "mother of the heart." The Native American tribe Flambeau Ojibwas reportedly used the berries and bark for "women's medicine."

Parts used
Flowers, leaves, and berries.

Active constituents
Amines (flowers only), flavonoids, phenolic acids, tannins, ascorbic acid.

How it works in the body
Hawthorn acts on the cardiovascular system, regulating the heartbeat, relaxing the arteries, and normalizing blood pressure—both lowering high blood pressure and raising low blood pressure. It can be used in angina and coronary artery disease to improve the bloodflow to the heart muscles. These medicinal benefits are thought to be due to a combination of the amines and the flavonoids. Its effects are not instant, but taken over a period of months hawthorn will reduce symptoms and act as a tonic to the heart. Chinese usage in the digestive system suggests the use of hawthorn to ease digestion of meat and greasy foods, and where there is pain, distension, and diarrhea. Chinese properties are sour, sweet, and slightly warm.

Applications
An infusion of the flowers, leaves, or berries may be taken, 200 ml (8 fl oz), three times a day on a long-term basis. The tincture may be taken 2–3 ml (40–60 drops), twice a day. There are no adverse effects from long-term use, and discontinuing use will produce no ill-effects. In Chinese medicine the dosage is 9–15 g (½–¾ oz).

Indications
- Symptoms of angina.
- Low or high blood pressure to restore to normal levels.
- Normalize an irregular heartbeat.
- Congestive heart failure and cardiomyopathy.

Contraindications
Do not discontinue or reduce orthodox medication for any cardiovascular condition without professional supervision. If you are receiving such medication you must consult an orthodox or herbal practitioner before using hawthorn. Chinese cautions indicate avoidance in cases of acid regurgitation.

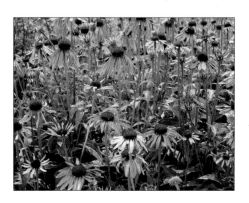

PURPLE CONE FLOWER

Compositae ECHINACEA PURPUREA/ANGUSTIFOLIA

This plant is native to North America, but is rapidly being cultivated in Europe and elsewhere in the world as its properties become recognized. The herb is distinctive, its name arising from the flower, which is shaped like a daisy, with a ring of purple florets around a central cone. The leaves are coarse and hairy.

History

The name derives from the Greek *echin*, or "hedgehog," referring to the prickly-looking central cone, which does resemble a hedgehog. The herb has also been called snake bite by Native Americans, who have used it for its ability to counter infection and also for bites from snakes and rabid animals. This information was passed to the early settlers, who continued to use it in a similar manner. Current research has certainly confirmed its ability to fight against infection through its antibacterial action, and has explored its role in improving and healing the immune system, especially where viral illnesses have taken hold, for example, in cases of chronic fatigue syndrome and AIDS. According to Vogel, *Echinacea* was burned by some Native Americans as a treatment for headaches, and also used as a remedy for toothache.

Parts used

Root, rhizome.

Active constituents

Echinacoside (only in *purpurea*), isobutyl amides (including echinacin), polysaccharides, polyacetylenes, essential oil, alkaloids, and flavonoids.

How it works in the body

The research into how *Echinacea* works on the immune system is continuing, but it is clear that the polysaccharides play a key role in preventing viruses from taking hold in the body's cells. In particular the herb stimulates the white T-cells within the immune system, which fight off infection and keep the body healthy. Of the other constituents, the alkaloids perform an antibacterial function, and are also active against fungal infection. It is also used as an alterative, or blood cleanser, for the skin, clearing boils and other skin complaints.

Applications

The herb is mainly used as a decoction of the root. For infections, both viral and bacterial, take 200 ml (8 fl oz), twice a day. As a tincture, take 2½ ml (50 drops/ ½ tsp) three times a day. For sore throats and mouth ulcers, combine 2 ml (40 drops) of the tincture with 2 ml (40 drops) marigold tincture and 2 ml (40 drops) myrrh tincture in 100 ml (4 fl oz) water, and gargle three times a day.

Indications

- Colds, flu, sore throats.
- Chronic fatigue syndrome.
- HIV and AIDS.
- Bacterial infections.
- Fungal infections such as candida (thrush).
- Skin complaints, including boils, acne, and eczema.
- Allergic conditions.

Contraindications

In order to get the best effect from its properties, it has been suggested that in cases of HIV and AIDS it is better to take *Echinacea* only for periods of three months at a time, and to alternate this with other immune system herbal remedies for about the same period.

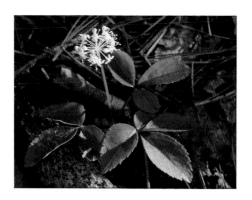

GINSENG

Araliaceae ELEUTHEROCCOCCUS SENTICOUS (*ren shen*)

Chinese pharmaceutical name: *radix ginseng*

There are three main types of ginseng—Siberian, panax, and American—which all belong to the same botanical family. The medicinal benefits are similar, but all three are looked at here. A native of Russia, China, Korea, and Japan, the ginseng bush grows to approximately three meters (9 ft). The American ginseng is native to North America and the Himalayas.

History

Russian research on Siberian ginseng has shown that its properties increase stamina and resistance to flus and other viruses. Panax ginseng has been used to improve athletic performance, and is given to improve virility in men.

Parts used

Root.

Active constituents

Siberian ginseng contains saponins, including eleutherosides A–F, glycans, volatile oil and two acetylenic compounds. Panax ginseng has saponin glycosides. American ginseng includes steroidal saponins.

How it works in the body

Siberian ginseng, more stimulating to the body than panax ginseng, helps increase stamina especially when under stress. It supports the adrenal glands, which produce hormones that are responsible for repair and growth. American ginseng is very similar to panax ginseng, but milder. In Chinese terms, panax ginseng is particularly indicated for shock where there is collapse of the *qi*, or energy. It is also used for shock where there is loss of blood. In lung conditions it is used for wheezing and shortness of breath in exertion brought on by lung *qi* deficiency. It is used to treat lethargy, lack of appetite, chest and abdominal distension, chronic diarrhea and, in severe cases, prolapse of the stomach, uterus, or rectum. It benefits the heart *qi*, calms the spirit, and helps palpitations with anxiety, insomnia, forgetfulness, and restlessness.

Applications

Make a decoction of the root and take 100 ml (4 fl oz) twice a day. The tincture may be taken 2 ml (40 drops) three times a day. Tablets are available commercially; follow the instructions given. The Chinese dosage is 1–9 g (¹⁄₁₆–½ oz). Because of its cost, the herb is usually decocted separately in small amounts of water in a double boiler (*see* Chinese herbal decoctions, p.32).

Indications

- Flus, colds, viral illnesses.
- Emotional and physical stress.
- Panax ginseng for male fertility problems.

Contraindications

Do not take for longer than four weeks at any one time. Ginseng should not be taken by those who are fit and healthy. Do not combine with other energy stimulants, such as coffee or guarana, as this will over-stress the system. Over-use of this herb may cause headaches; stick to the recommended dosage. **Do not** take during pregnancy or while breastfeeding. **Do not** give to children under the age of 12. Chinese cautions indicate it should not be taken with high blood pressure. It should only be used with signs of weakness. Over-dosage of this herb may also cause insomnia and palpitations. The traditional antidote is mung bean soup.

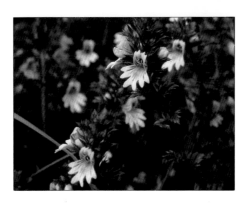

EYEBRIGHT

Scrophulariaceae EUPHRASIA OFFICINALIS

Eyebright is one of a family of *Euphrasias* growing in Europe, Asia, and North America. It grows on dry and chalky ground, but on rich soil can grow to about 25 cm (10 in). It is a semiparasite, dependent on roots of grass from which it draws nutrients, without damaging the grass itself. The leaves are oval, and the flowers, appearing in summer, are white or lilac, shot through with purple veins.

History

The name *Euphrasia* comes from the Greek *Euphrossyne*, or gladness, which was the name of one of the Three Graces. Gladness is associated with the happiness of the person whose eyesight is benefited by the plant. Another tradition is that *Euphrasia* is also the name given to the Linnet, who used the leaves to clear the sight of her young, and gave the knowledge to humans who named the plant in her honor. There is no mention of its use, however, before the 14th century, but in the 17th century it was used as a wine, and in Queen Elizabeth's time as an ale.

Parts used

Whole herb.

Active constituents

Iridoid glycosides, tannins, phenolic acids, volatile oils, alkaloids, sterols.

How it works in the body

The astringent qualities found in eyebright form a protective layer on the mucous membranes of the eyes and so reduce inflammation. This is especially beneficial for infections such as conjunctivitis. In addition, it is helpful where there is an allergic condition, such as the streaming or irritated eyes which occur with hayfever, or the effects of pollution.

Applications

As an infusion, eyebright tea may be taken internally three times a day to counter infection or allergic conditions, especially where there is watering of the eyes. Externally, it may be used either as a compress or an eyebath for sore or irritated eyes. The eyebath should not be used more than twice a day. Carefully follow the instructions in the Herbal Methods section (*see* p.22) for preparations concerning the eyes.

Indications

- Infections or inflammations of the eye such as conjunctivitis and blephiritis.
- Allergic conditions including hayfever and allergic rhinitis.
- Tired or reddened eyes due to overwork, pollution, and tiredness.

Contraindications

For any eye condition which does not resolve in three to four days, seek further advice from a qualified herbal or medical practitioner. For any sudden pain or loss of vision in the eyes, seek medical help immediately.

Benefits of eyebright

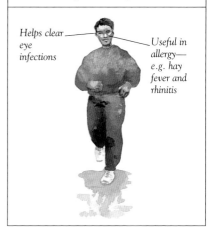

Helps clear eye infections

Useful in allergy— e.g. hay fever and rhinitis

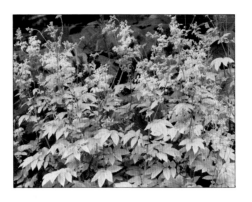

MEADOWSWEET

Rosaceae FILIPENDULA ULMARIA

Native to Europe, Britain, and parts of Asia, this meadow plant is also naturalized in North America. It grows to about 1½ meters (5 ft). Its paired and toothed leaves are green on top and pale underneath, with clusters of creamy flowers and a delicious scent. It prefers damp conditions, often on riverbanks.

History

The flower blooms from June to September, giving off an almond-like scent. It was used in the Middle Ages as a strewing herb to freshen the staleness of the atmosphere in churches and other public places. Gerard wrote that the scent, "makes the heart merrie and joyful and delighteth the senses." The herb was often added to beer or wine and was used to make a type of mead in Chaucer's time. The name *ulmaria* is given in reference to the leaves which resemble those of the elm (*ulmus*) tree. A decoction of the root in wine was considered specific in the treatment of fevers. Meadowsweet, verbena, and water-mint were three herbs held to be most sacred by the Druids. During the 19th century, the salicylic component of meadowsweet was the original substance extracted to create aspirin. The plant's natural balancers mean that is does not have any of the side-effects of the synthesized drug, such as gastric bleeding.

Parts used
Flowering herb, including leaves.

Active constituents
Volatile oil, with salicylaldehyde; phenolic glycosides, flavonoids, polyphenolics, tannins, coumarin, ascorbic acid.

How it works in the body
The salicylic component is responsible for the action of the plant as an anti-inflammatory and painkiller, used in musculoskeletal disorders, such as arthritis. It is this constituent which is used in the digestive system in conditions of excess acidity, for example, where there is indigestion caused by the over-production of acid, stomach ulcers, and in irritable bowel syndrome. It is not merely thought to reduce acidity, but to actively promote healing in the gut where there is inflammation. It has long been used as a gentle remedy for diarrhea, and extolled as a specific for children's diarrhea, which is endorsed by medical herbalists today.

Applications
Use as an infusion, 200 ml (8 fl oz) three times a day for digestive disorders, use a double-strength infusion and take three times a day for diarrhea in adults. Take the tincture, 2 ml (40 drops) three times a day for arthritis complaints.

Indications
• Digestive complaints, especially with acidity, for example, gastric ulcers, irritable bowel syndrome.
• Diarrhea in adults and children.
• Arthritis complaints.

Contraindications
Do not take where there is sensitivity to salicylates, or allergy to aspirin.

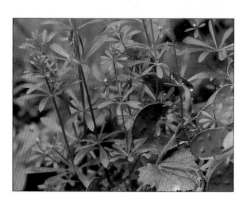

CLEAVERS

Rubiaceae GALIUM APARINE

A garden weed, with long, thin stems and rings or whorls of leaves covered in tiny prickles which catch on clothing, animals, or other plants. The whole plant grows to about 1½ meters (4 ft), and twines itself round and through other plants. The flowers are tiny, white or greenish white, and star-like. It grows throughout Europe and North America, in hedges and waste grounds.

History

Many of the common names of this plant describe its clinging nature: cleavers, catchweed, and ever-lasting friendship. The official name, *galium aparine*, is derived from the Greek, *galium* meaning "milk," and *aparine* from *aparo*, or "to seize." The reference to milk refers to its reputed use as an agent to curdle milk, while "to seize" refers again to its tenacious character. The seeds, dried and slightly roasted, were used as a substitute for coffee in Sweden. The stems of the whole plant have been reportedly used in Greece and Sweden as a sieve for milk. It is said that the roots when eaten by birds tend to tinge their bones red. It used to be a favorite ingredient in the old spring tonics made after long winters when fresh greens were just reappearing and was often used in country areas as a cold remedy.

Parts used

Leaves and stems.

Active constituents

Iridoids, polyphenolic acids, anthra-quinones (roots), alkanes and flavonoids, tannins and coumarins.

How it works in the body

Cleavers' main action is that of a diuretic. As a way of eliminating toxins from the body via the urinary system, it is used for kidney stones and other urinary com-plaints, such as cystitis. In addition, its eliminative nature means it is helpful in skin conditions, e.g., eczema and psoriasis. It is thought to be an effective lymphatic cleanser, and is used in swollen lymph glands. It is possibly a combination of these detoxifying properties that has promoted its use in cancers and similar illnesses. One of the iridoids acts as a mild laxative. There is some research into its properties with regard to the lowering of blood pressure. It has reportedly been used for insomnia.

Applications

As a juice taken internally, it is reportedly at its best for cases of swellings and tumors. Wash the fresh herb and add it with water to a food processor, or blender to pulp it. Strain the juice and drink a wineglassful a day. It is possible to freeze the juice in icetrays, and defrost as required. Externally, it has been used as a cream or ointment for lumps and ulcerations. Internally, as an infusion take 1 cup, 200 ml (8 fl oz), three times a day. Externally, the cooled infusion may be used as a wash or poultice for inflamed skin conditions.

Indications

- Internally, skin conditions such as eczema and psoriasis.
- Externally, ulcerations and tumors.
- Urinary tract complaints, such as kidney stones and cystitis.
- For the nervous system as a sleep tonic.
- Swollen lymph glands.

Contraindications

Do not use if there is low blood pressure.

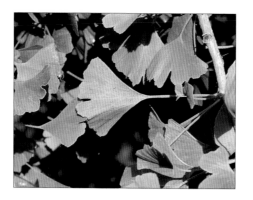

GINKGO

Ginkgoaceae GINKGO BILOBA (*bai guo*)

Also known as the maidenhair tree, ginkgo is a giant fern, native to China and Japan. It has one or more trunks, and the leaves are notable for their fan-like shape.

History

Ginkgo is thought to be the oldest living species of tree, with some trees known to live for 1,000 years. It was the only growing plant to survive Hiroshima. It has been used as a remedy in China for thousands of years. With research currently confirming its use as an agent to improve declining mental faculties, ginkgo is becoming increasingly popular—so much so that it may possibly become endangered.

Parts used

Leaves and seeds.

Active constituents

Lignans; the ginkgolides (A, B and C), flavonoids, terpenes, essential oil, tannins.

How it works in the body

The ginkgolides, especially B, work as a platelet activating factor (PAF) antagonist. PAF is involved in initiating both allergic and inflammatory reactions, and in particular asthma. The flavonoid portion is the agent thought to improve circulation to the brain.

Applications

Leaves are prepared as an infusion; take 200 ml (8 fl oz) twice a day. Seeds are used as a decoction, again, take 200 ml (8 fl oz) twice a day. Tincture is prepared from the leaves, and for circulatory problems should be taken 5 ml (1 tsp), three times a day. Tablets are available commercially. Treatment needs to last at least three months to affect improvement in mental faculties. Chinese dosage for the leaves is 3–6 g (⅛–¼ oz) and the dosage for the seed is 4.5–9 g (¼–½ oz).

Indications

• Circulation, to aid memory, concentration, and age-related dementia.
• Asthma, particularly in children (only use under the guidance of a medical or herbal practitioner).

Contraindications

Before using ginkgo consult a herbal or medical practitioner if you are already taking medication for a circulatory-related condition. In asthma cases, **do not** discontinue orthodox medications, and consult a herbal or medical practitioner before using herbal remedies. **Do not** exceed the dose stated, as large amounts can cause adverse reactions. In Chinese medicine, this herb is considered slightly toxic, and should only be used in small amounts for short periods of time under a qualified practitioner. Symptoms of overdose include headache, tremors, fever, and irritability. The antidote is 60 g (3 oz) of Radix Glycyrrhizae Uralensis (*gan cao*) or 30 g (1½ oz) of boiled ginkgo shells.

Benefits of ginkgo

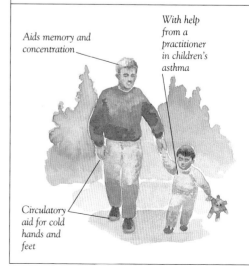

Aids memory and concentration

With help from a practitioner in children's asthma

Circulatory aid for cold hands and feet

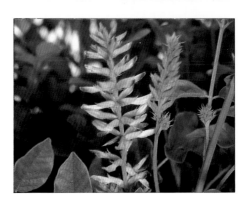

LICORICE

Leguminosae GLYCYRRHIZA GLABRA (*gan cao*)

A native of southern Europe and Asia, licorice has many different species. Although most have roots which possess a degree of sweetness, few are exceptionally sweet and also possess medicinal value. It grows to about two meters (6 ft) and has pale-yellow flowers.

History

Licorice was mentioned by the Greeks in the third century BC. The name is from the Greek *glucos*, meaning sweet, and *riza*, meaning root. Licorice comes from the Latin *liquiritia*. It was in common use in Germany in the Middle Ages, and was cultivated in England in 1562.

Parts used

Root.

Active constituents

Triterpenes (mainly glycyrrhizin), flavonoids and isoflavonoids, coumarins, chalcones, polysaccharides, volatile oil, starch, sugars.

How it works in the body

The glycyrrhizin, which is 50 times sweeter than sugar, is mainly responsible for the plant's function in the respiratory system, acting as an expectorant and helping to prevent and ease coughing. This ingredient and its derivatives work as an anti-inflammatory. It is also largely the glycyrrhizin which gives an anti-allergenic effect, especially when treating asthma. In the digestive system, licorice is known to have a protective effect on the liver, helping to detoxify and rid the body of unwanted elements. In China it has been used to treat hepatitis and jaundice. The plant is also used to treat nausea, bloating, and vomiting, and is a valuable agent for the treatment of stomach ulcers. Licorice has a beneficial effect on the adrenal glands, supporting them in their function of healing the body. The herb also has immuno-stimulant properties, and possibly anticarcinogenic principles. It is also available as a commercially-prepared extract which is called "deglycyrrhizinated licorice" or "DGL." American research found DGL to be effective in the treatment of ulcers and less likely to raise blood pressure. As DGL is commercially prepared it is not strictly a home herbal remedy. Licorice obtained and prepared at home should still be regarded with caution since it should not be taken in conditions of high blood pressure. Chinese properties are sweet and neutral if used raw; sweet and warming if dry-fried before using in a decoction.

Applications

As a decoction, take 100 ml (4 fl oz) daily for constipation. Take as a tincture, 2 ml (40 drops) twice a day for all other complaints. Make as a syrup to ease sore throats and dry coughs. The Chinese dosage is 2–12 g (⅛–⅜ oz).

Indications

- Bloating, nausea, indigestion, and also stomach ulcers.
- A gentle laxative.
- Mouthwash for mouth ulcers.
- For dry coughs, and as an expectorant for catarrhal conditions.
- For mild asthma (under the supervision of a qualified medical or herbal practitioner).
- Chest complaints, including bronchitic conditions.
- Arthritis, where there are inflamed joints.
- To support the adrenal glands.

Contraindications

Licorice should **not** be taken during pregnancy. **Do not** take if suffering from high blood pressure.

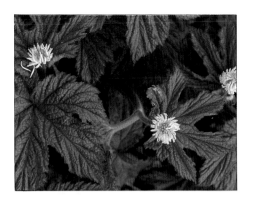

GOLDENSEAL

Ranunculaceae HYDRASTIS CANADENSIS

A native of Canada and the eastern United States, this herb from the buttercup family grows to about 15–30 cm (6–12 in). The hairy stem leads to two lobed leaves and a small greenish-white flower. It has red fruit and a yellow root.

History

Commonly known as yellow root, or yellow puccoon by Native Americans, there was confusion as to the exact species as these were also names given to other plants. It was used as a remedy by the Cherokees and later by settlers, but was not recognized medicinally officially until about 1798.

Parts used

Rhizome.

Active constituents

Isoquinoline alkaloids (including hydrastine, berberine and canadine), fatty acids, resin, polyphenolic acids, volatile oil.

How it works in the body

The isoquinoline alkaloids are thought to be largely responsible for goldenseal's medicinal actions, the hydrastine acting as an astringent and as a hemostatic agent (stops bleeding). The berberine has both antibacterial and amoebicidal properties, while the canadine is thought to stimulate the uterine muscles. Goldenseal's main use is in the treatment of mucous membranes throughout the body. It is used in the respiratory system for conditions of excess mucus and also for the eyes, nose, and throat where inflammation is present. Its antibacterial properties make it useful for infection, especially in the mouth or eyes. Used for short periods of time as a tonic it can increase appetite and stimulate the digestion. In the reproductive system it alleviates heavy bleeding and astringes the membranes where there is vaginal infection.

Applications

As a decoction, goldenseal may be used as a gargle or mouthwash, two or three times a day. The powder may be prepared as an infusion for use as a douche in cases of vaginal infections. The tincture may be taken 1 ml (20 drops), twice daily. A dilute infusion may be used as an eyewash.

Indications

- Sore throats (gargle); sore gums, mouth ulcers (mouthwash).
- Inflamed or sore eyes (eyewash).
- Stimulate the appetite (tonic).
- Mild laxative (with other herbs).
- Reduces heavy menstrual bleeding.

Contraindications

Do not take in pregnancy or while breastfeeding as it is a uterine stimulant. **Do not** take in high blood pressure. **Do not** exceed the dosages stated as goldenseal is toxic in large amounts.

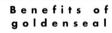

Benefits of goldenseal

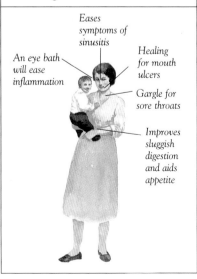

Eases symptoms of sinusitis

Healing for mouth ulcers

An eye bath will ease inflammation

Gargle for sore throats

Improves sluggish digestion and aids appetite

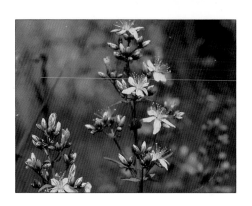

ST JOHN'S WORT

Hypericaceae HYPERICUM PERFOLIATUM

This plant is native to Europe and Britain, but grows in many other parts of the world and has been imported to thrive in North America. It can grow to about one meter (3 ft) high, and has small green leaves and bright-yellow flowers with five petals. The petals of the flowers have small black dots on the margin underneath, which are in fact oil glands.

History

The name *Hypericum* comes from the Greek *hyper*, meaning over, and *erico*, an apparition, which is a reference to its reputation for driving out evil spirits. St John's wort is so-called because it is believed to flower first on St John's Day, the 24th of June. In studies it has been shown that when compared alongside orthodox antidepressants in trials, St John's wort has a comparable beneficial effect, with fewer side-effects. Note: Caution is required as American research has found that some people experienced hyperactivity or numbness in the hands. Its value as an immune-system herb is being harnessed in conditions such as HIV and other viral illnesses, and research into this is continuing.

Parts used

Whole herb.

Active constituents

Essential oil, hypericins, flavonoids, and epicatechin.

How it works in the body

St John's wort works primarily in the nervous system, the hypericin in combination with the other constituents acting as an anti-depressant. American studies have found that this herb may be used in combination with *Ginkgo biloba* to increase antidepressant effectiveness. However, if you wish to combine these herbs, or are already taking prescription antidepressants, it is advisable to first consult your medical or herbal practitioner. St John's wort is also a tonic for the nervous system as a whole, and can be used, for example, in the reproductive system in menopause, where physical changes are aggravated by mental and emotional debility. In the digestive system, the herb is beneficial to the liver, and in the respiratory system, the antiviral properties make it especially useful in colds and flus. Its antiviral benefits are used to improve the immune system as a whole. Externally, the oil is used as an antiseptic to heal wounds and to ease nerve pain, for example, in shingles and repetitive strain injury.

Applications

As an infusion, take 200 ml (8 fl oz), twice a day. The tincture should be taken 2 ml (40 drops), three times a day. Externally, the oil may be applied twice a day (*see* Herbal Methods, nerve tonic oil, p.25). As a cream, apply twice a day to stings or cuts.

Indications

- Anti-depressant.
- Nervous system tonic.
- Menopause associated with emotional debility.
- Tonic for the digestive system.
- Colds and flu.
- Viral complaints, such as herpes, HIV, and AIDS.
- Topically, for shingles and repetitive strain injury.
- For stings or cuts.

Contraindications

Do not exceed the stated dosage. Over-use of this herb can cause photosensitivity in some people.

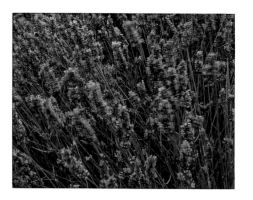

LAVENDER

Labiatae LAVANDULA OFFICINALIS/ANGUSTIFOLIA

This well-known shrub is native to the western Mediterranean, and cultivated in many other countries for its fragrance, which has been used in cosmetics. There are many different species. The leaves are narrow, gray-green, and the flowers form a pale to dark purple spike at the end of a tall stalk. It grows to about one meter (3 ft) in height.

History

Used by the Romans as a perfume for the bath, the plant possibly derived its name from *lavare* which is the Latin word for "to wash." It was introduced in England in about 1568 and taken to America by the Pilgrims. In Portugal and Spain it was used as a strewing herb for scenting churches on important occasions, and was also burnt to keep evil spirits away. In the Middle Ages it was one of the ingredients of four thieves' vinegar, used by grave robbers to ward off the plague. In Gerard's time, lavender was used as a flavoring for food, and conserves of lavender were said to comfort the stomach, while the tea was recommended to relieve headache and exhaustion.

Parts used

Flowers, essential oil.

Active constituents

Volatile oil, coumarins, triterpenes.

How it works in the body

Lavender has a calming and relaxing quality which makes it suitable for use in the body's many systems. Lavender is helpful in the digestive system, where it is used to calm indigestion and related symptoms such as wind and bloating. In the nervous system, it is used for headaches, depression, and sleeplessness. It is also used in asthma, where there is a nervous element contributing to the symptoms. Topically, it is added to creams and oils as a rub in arthritic complaints, as it acts as a painkiller relieving painful joints. For neuralgia or nerve pain, it is useful externally in creams and oils.

Applications

For indigestion, as an infusion, take 100 ml (4 fl oz) twice daily. For sleeplessness, as a tincture take 3–5 ml (½–1 tsp) at night. Add lavender infusion or essential oil to a bath before bedtime to relieve stress and tension, or use in a diffuser to aid sleep. For headaches, add two drops of lavender essential oil to a bowl of cold water and soak a cloth to make a compress to place across the forehead. Five drops of lavender oil added to a footbath relieves exhaustion. As a rub for arthritic complaints add one drop each of lavender essential oil and wintergreen essential oil to 50 ml (4 tbsp) of a carrier oil. You may use the essential oil neat on insect bites or stings.

Indications

- Indigestion, wind, and bloating.
- Insomnia.
- Nervous complaints, including stress, tension, headaches.
- Arthritic complaints.
- Neuralgia.
- Insect bites and stings.

Contraindications

Never take essential oils internally. Do not add them to a baby's bath as it can ingest the oils from its hands.

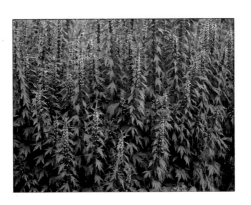

MOTHERWORT
Labiatae LEONURUS CARDIACA (*yi mu cao*)
Chinese pharmaceutical name: *herba leonuri heterophylli*

A native of Europe, this plant grows to about one meter (3 ft), with dull-green, hairy leaves, and clusters of pink flowers. It is naturalized in other countries, including England and North America. It grows mainly on wasteground, but is occasionally cultivated in gardens. Another variety, *Leonurus hetrophyllus*, is used in Chinese herbalism in the same way as *cardiaca*.

History

The name *Leonurus* is from the Greek meaning "lion's tail," and *cardiaca*, which refers to the heart. This name indicates its traditional use as a herbal remedy for palpitations, especially of a nervous origin. In old herbals it has often been referred to as a tonic to both strengthen the heart and to relieve stress placed on the heart by nervous disorders. Culpeper wrote, ". . . there is no better herb to drive melancholy vapours from the heart."

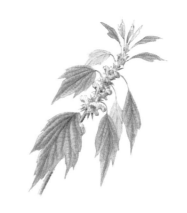

Parts used
Whole herb.

Active constituents
Iridoids, diterpenes, flavonoids, caffeic acid.

How it works in the body

As its history indicates, motherwort is a remedy for the cardiovascular system, particularly where there are palpitations and when they are aggravated by nervous tension or stress. Its actions are antispasmodic and sedative, helping to regulate the heart, and also acting as a tonic to strengthen weakness of the heart. It can be used where there is high blood pressure. In addition, in the reproductive system, it helps to bring on a delayed period by stimulating the uterine muscles. It is also used where there is premenstrual syndrome, especially in early menopause. In Chinese herbalism, its use in the reproductive system extends from irregular periods and premenstrual pain, to a treatment for infertility and immobile abdominal masses. The Chinese properties are acrid, bitter, and slightly cold.

Applications
Take an infusion, 200 ml (8 fl oz), twice daily. For the tincture, take 2 ml (40 drops), three times a day. The Chinese dosage is 9–60 g (½–3 oz).

Indications
- Palpitations associated with nervous tension and stress.
- Tonic for the heart.
- High blood pressure.
- PMS, especially in menopause.

Contraindications
Do not take motherwort during pregnancy. This is confirmed in Chinese cautions. Do not take in reproductive conditions where there is a tendency to heavy periods.

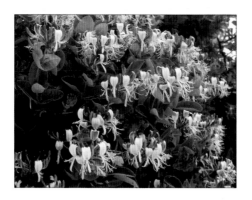

HONEYSUCKLE

Caprifoliaceae LONICERA SPECIES *(jin yin hua)*

Chinese pharmaceutical name: *flos lonicerae japonicae*

Honeysuckle is a European native, but is grown extensively throughout the world, especially in China, and there are many varieties. In Europe the most common is *Lonicera caprifolium*, while in China it is *Lonicera japonica*. It is a climbing shrub, growing to some four meters (12 ft). It has oval leaves which grow opposite each other, and yellow flowers either tinged with orange (*caprifolium*) or white (*japonica*). The flowers give way to red berries.

History

Culpeper said, "The leaves, which are the only part used, are sometimes put into gargarisms for sore throats . . . Some command a decoction of them for a cough." The herbalist Gerard wrote in the 16th century, "The floures steeped in oile and set in the Sun, are good to annoint the body that is benummed, and growne very cold." The family name *Lonicera* was given by Linnaeus, the Swedish botanist who originated the system of botanical naming, in honor of Adam Lonicer, who wrote many botanical books. The *Lonicera japonica* was first mentioned in the *Tang Materia Medica*.

Parts used
Flowers and leaves.

Active constituents
Volatile oil, luteolin, inositol, tannins.

How it works in the body
Western applications of *Lonicera caprifolium* tend to follow the age-old usage, that is, the leaves are used as a gargle or mouthwash for sore throats and gum problems, while the flowers are commonly used in treatments for asthma, where they relax the airways. The Chinese usage of *Lonicera japonica* is much more extensive, and research has shown an antibacterial action against both *streptococcus* and *staphylococcus* bacteria. In laboratory experiments, some protective effects on the lungs have been demonstrated in cases of tuberculosis. Traditional Chinese applications include cases of abscesses or swellings, especially of the breast, throat, eyes, or internally. It is also used in the early stages of diseases accompanied by fever, sensitivity to wind, sore throat, and headache. It is also used in cases of damp-heat dysenteric

disorders, or painful urinary dysfunction. The Chinese properties are sweet and cold.

Applications
Use as an infusion 200 ml (8 fl oz), twice daily, internally. Use the infusion as a gargle or mouthwash, twice daily (*see* Herbal Methods, gargles and mouthwashes, p.21). Chinese dosage is 9–15 g (½–¾ oz).

Indications
- Sore throats and gum problems.
- Asthma (under the supervision of a qualified herbal or medicinal practitioner).
- Infections accompanied by fever, sore throat, headache.
- Abscesses or swellings, especially of the breast or throat.
- Dysentery or painful urinary dysfunction.

Contraindications
The berries should not be taken, as they are poisonous. The Chinese cautions indicate that this remedy should not be used in cases of diarrhea. It is also contraindicated for sores where there is *qi* (energy) deficiency, as demonstrated by a clear discharge.

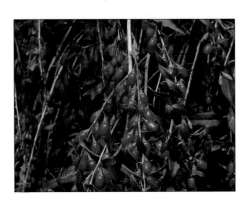

LYCIUM FRUIT

Solanaceae LYCIUM CHINENSE *(gou qi zi)*
Chinese pharmaceutical name: *fructus lycii*

This shrub is native to and cultivated widely throughout China. It grows to about four meters (12 feet) and displays distinctive, bright-red berries.

History

This plant first appeared medicinally in the *Divine Husbandman's Classic of the Materia Medica*, AD 1, and has been used for thousands of years. Research has shown that the herb has a protective effect on the liver, and also aids its recovery from the effects of toxicity. In laboratory conditions it was demonstrated to be effective in breaking down lipids. It has been further shown to lower blood pressure and ease breathing. In folk medicine it has been used for disorders where wasting and thirst are features. It is also known as Chinese wolfberry fruit and matrimony vine fruit.

Parts used

Berries and root.

Active constituents

Betaine, carotene, physalien, thiamine, riboflavine, vitamin C, beta-sitosterol, and linoleic acid.

How it works in the body

The berries are thought to have a protective effect on the liver and kidneys, nourishing and acting as a tonic. Conditions where this is most effective are those where there is a sore back and legs, low-grade abdominal pain, excessive urination at night (nocturia), wasting and thirsting disorders, consumption, and, in the reproductive system for men, impotence. Another of its major functions is as a tonic for the eyes, especially where the circulation is thought to be poor, in conditions of dizziness, blurred vision, and diminished sight. In the respiratory system it is used to tonify the lungs, especially in conditions with a consumptive cough. In the cardiovascular system it is used as a circulatory tonic, to reduce blood pressure and to lower lipid levels. The Chinese properties are those of sweet and neutral.

Applications

Both the berries and the root are made as a decoction, 200 ml (8 fl oz) a day. A tincture of the root can be made, take 5 ml (1 tsp), twice daily. The Chinese dosage is 6–18 g (⅛–⅛ oz).

Indications

- Tonic for the liver and kidney.
- Improves circulation, reduces high blood pressure, and lowers lipid levels.
- Where wasting and thirst are a feature, such as diabetes.
- Consumptive coughs.
- Tonic for the eyes.
- Tonic for male impotence.

Contraindications

Chinese cautions indicate that this herb should not be used in cases of digestive weakness where the stools are loose.

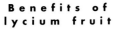

Benefits of lycium fruit

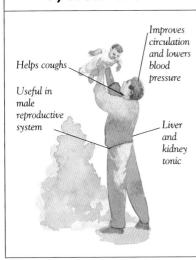

Improves circulation and lowers blood pressure

Helps coughs

Useful in male reproductive system

Liver and kidney tonic

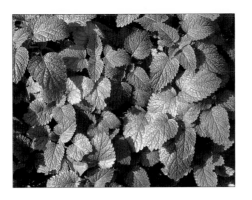

LEMON BALM

Labiatae MELISSA OFFICINALIS

Common in Europe, Britain, Asia, North Africa, and North America, lemon balm grows to about 1½ meters (5 ft) high. The oval leaves have serrated edges that occur in pairs along the stem. When crushed they emit a lemon aroma. The flowers are white, occurring in the axils of the leaves.

History
Lemon balm is a bee plant, the Greek name *Melissa* actually meaning bee. Balm comes from the word balsam, meaning "balm for your sorrows." Gerard said "It is profitably planted where bees are kept," while John Evelyn wrote, "Balm is sovereign for the brain, strengthening the memory and powerfully chasing away melancholy." Lemon balm, when combined with nutmeg, angelica, and lemon peel, was known as Carmelite water, and used as a remedy for nervous headaches and neuralgia.

Parts used
Leaves and flowers, essential oil.

Active constituents
Volatile oil, flavonoids, polyphenolics (including rosmarinic acid, triterpenic acids).

How it works in the body
In the nervous system, the oil is the main agent used to calm and soothe, and has a relaxant effect on the muscles. This has been supported by research, where melissa has been used in states of excitability, palpitations, depression, and headache. The polyphenolics, especially the rosmarinic acid, are responsible for an antiviral action: a cream made from lemon balm has been shown to be affective against herpes simplex, more commonly known as cold sores. The duration of the outbreaks have been halved and the outbreaks themselves become less frequent. Lemon balm also has an action on the thyroid by reducing over-activity of the gland (hyperthyroidism). In the reproductive system, this herb has been used in the menopause to ease symptoms, including hot flushes and anxiety, and to regulate periods, as well as alleviating period pains.

Applications
Use as an infusion, 200 ml (8 fl oz), three times a day in states of nervous excitability, headaches, etc. Use the tincture 3 ml (60 drops) twice a day internally for viral complaints. Prepare as a cream or ointment to use topically on cold sores (*see* Herbal Methods pp.26–27). Use the essential oil in an oil burner to uplift the spirits, or add to a bath to relieve stress and tension.

Indications
- Nervous complaints.
- Internally (tincture) for viral complaints, such as cold sores, shingles, colds and flu.
- Externally for cold sores.
- In menopause, to ease symptoms.
- To help regulate periods and alleviate period pain.

Contraindications
Do not use the oil internally. Do not add oil to a baby's bath as they can ingest the oil through their hands.

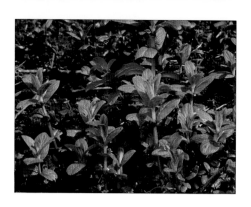

PEPPERMINT

Labiatae MENTHA PIPERITA *(bo he)*

Chinese pharmaceutical name: *herba menthae haplocalycis*

A native of Europe, mint is perhaps one of the best-known culinary herbs. The medicinal variety is a hybrid—a naturally occurring combination of watermint and spearmint. The plant is widely cultivated in many countries, and in particular in North America. The leaves are green with a serrated edge which give off the familiar mint odor when crushed between the fingers, and with small, reddish-purple flowers. It grows to about 40 cm (15 in) in height, and there are two types, the black and the white peppermint.

History
According to Vogel, wild mint was used by Missouri Valley tribes as a carminative, and among many others to alleviate fevers.

Parts used
Leaves, essential oil.

Active constituents
Essential oil, up to 1.5 per cent, containing menthol, flavonoids, rosmarinic acid.

How it works in the body
The menthol in the oil is responsible for an antiseptic effect on the body as a whole. The leaves, with their combination of constituents are useful in the treatment of digestive disorders, having an antispasmodic effect which is calming on the gut, especially where there is gastric upset due to over-indulgence. It is also used in complaints such as irritable bowel syndrome, gastritis, and where there is excess wind and colic. It has a diaphoretic element which encourages sweating, so has been used in colds and flu to cool down a fever. In Chinese terms it is also used to disperse fever, headaches, and coughs, and is used in the early stages of colds and flu. Additionally, the Chinese use it for rashes, for example in measles, as it encourages the rash to progress and thereby speeds recovery. It can also act as a painkiller, when applied externally. The oil has antibacterial properties. The Chinese properties are those of acrid, aromatic, and cooling.

Applications
As an infusion, 200 ml (8 fl oz) of peppermint can be taken three times a day, after meals to aid the digestion. In colds and flu, add a pinch of the herb to a tea made of equal parts of yarrow and elderflower to relieve symptoms. Take as a tincture, 1 ml (20 drops), three times a day for digestive problems. Externally use 10 drops of the oil in 50 ml (4 tbsp) of carrier oil to rub on to inflamed joints. Peppermint capsules are available on prescription only—**do not** take the oil internally. The Chinese dosage is 1.5–6 g (¹⁄₁₆– ¼ oz). Add to the decoction five minutes before finishing; it must not be overcooked.

Indications
- Irritable bowel syndrome, gastritis, excess wind, and colic.
- Colds and flu—add a pinch to other herbal remedies to help reduce a fever.
- Externally, use the oil to relieve the plain of inflamed joints.

Contraindications
Do not give peppermint to children under 12, either as an infusion, or the essential oil topically. **Do not** take the essential oil internally. The Chinese cautions recommend this herb not be given to nursing mothers as it may stem milkflow. Also, take care in weakness or prolonged fevers.

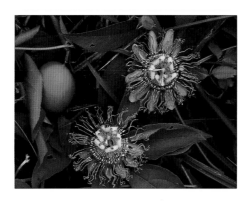

PASSION FLOWER

Passifloraceae PASSIFLORA INCARNATA

Passion flower is native to the southern United States and also to central and South America. It is cultivated in many countries. It is a climber, of approximately nine meters (30 ft) in length, with curling tendrils and striking flowers, with pale petals with purple fronds within which gives way to large, oval, orange berries. It grows in sunny positions where there is rich soil. There are many different varieties.

History

The name passion flower refers to the Passion or Crucifixion of Christ in the Christian tradition. The flower's central corona is thought to resemble Christ's crown of thorns, while the five stamens are linked to the five wounds, and the three styles to the nails. It was listed in the herbals of the Aztecs as an emetic and purgative, and the Mayas used it for swellings and for ringworm. It has been used for epilepsy. Native Americans traditionally used it for sedative qualities for restlessness, insomnia, and in the treatment of neuralgia.

Parts used

Leaves.

Active constituents

Alkaloids (some of which have not been fully verified), flavonoids (including apigenin, an 8-pyrone derivative), sterols, and sugars.

How it works in the body

Passiflora is primarily a sedative acting on the central nervous system, through the combined actions of the alkaloids, flavonoids, and the 8-pyrone derivative, although the mechanisms by which this works are not extensively researched as yet. Its sedative qualities have been used in overactive states ranging from epilepsy to neuralgia and anxiety. It is extremely useful in states of sleeplessness. One flavonoid, apigenin, is known to have antispasmodic and anti-inflammatory action which has been used in the cardiovascular system, to ease high blood pressure, and quiet palpitations. In other systems it is used to ease muscle spasm.

Applications

As an infusion, take 200–400 ml (8–16 fl oz) daily. As a tincture take 2 ml (40 drops) three times a day, or 5 ml (1 tsp) at night for insomnia. This herb is also available commercially as tablets.

Indications

- Insomnia.
- Anxiety, states of restlessness, panic attacks.
- Neuralgia as a mild painkiller.
- High blood pressure.
- Relaxant in diverticulitis and irritable bowel syndrome.
- To relax the airways.
- Period and ovarian pain.

Contraindications

Do not use during pregnancy. Large doses can lead to a soporific state.

Benefits of passion flower

Useful in insomnia

Relieves anxiety and panic attacks

Relaxes digestion in irritable bowel syndrome

Mild painkiller for neuralgia

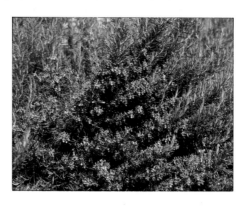

ROSEMARY

Labiatae ROSMARINUS OFFICINALIS

A native of the Mediterranean regions, this plant is well known as a culinary herb, and cultivated widely in gardens in many parts of the world. It grows as a shrub to about two meters (6 ft) high, with woody stems and narrow, needle-like leaves. The flowers are tiny, pale lilac, or blue. The scent is distinctive.

History

Rosemary has a long history for improving the memory. It was often used as a floral emblem of love and fidelity for this reason, being included in a wedding bouquet. Sir Thomas More wrote, "I lett it runne all over my garden walls, not onlie because my bees love it, but because it is the herb sacred to remembrance and, therefore, to friendship." It also has a tradition of being grown in gardens where the woman ruled the household. Rosemary has been burnt as an incense to cleanse the air in sickrooms, and was placed, together with rue, in courtrooms to offset contagion from prisoners held in the jails. The name *Rosmarinus* comes from the Latin meaning dew of the sea, a reference to its refreshing effect on the spirit.

Parts used

Leaves, essential oil.

Active constituents

Volatile oil, flavonoids, including apigenin and diosmetin, rosmarinic acid and other phenolic acids, diterpenes, triterpenes, including ursolic acid.

How it works in the body

One of rosemary's primary actions is that of an anti-inflammatory and tonic, which is thought to be due to combined constituents, including the apigenin, rosmarinic, and ursolic acids. The diosmetin is known to help in strengthening the capillaries, which is valuable in the cardiovascular system, where rosemary is used to improve circulation and raise low blood pressure. This circulatory effect is particularly directed at the circulation to the head, which is thought to contribute to improving the memory and concentration. It is also used where there is Reynaud's Syndrome, a condition of poor circulation in the hands and feet. It is also used where there is listlessness and depression, and for that reason can improve states of lethargy and debility.

Applications

The infusion can be taken 200 ml (8 fl oz) daily, internally. Externally, use the infusion as a rinse for the hair to improve circulation to the scalp. It can also be added to the bath as a refreshing way to start the day. The tincture can be taken, 2 ml (40 drops), twice a day. The essential oil can be added to bathwater or used in a diffuser, and is helpful for concentration and to aid studying.

Indications

- Improves circulation to the brain to aid memory and concentration.
- Cold hands and feet.
- Low blood pressure.
- States of debility.
- As a hair rinse to improve the scalp and encourage hair growth.

Contraindications

This herb should not be used in high blood pressure.

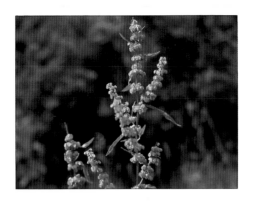

YELLOW DOCK

Polygonaceae RUMEX CRISPUS

Also commonly called curled dock, this refers to the shape of the leaves, which are large and similar to other docks except with regard to the extremely furled edges. It is largely found in wastelands and by the side of roads. Its origins are Europe and Africa, but is now transplanted to many other parts of the world.

History

This herb, along with others in the same species, is known for its cleansing properties. Long used as a way of ridding the system of toxins, Culpeper recommended it for expelling damaging "cholers" from the body. He went on to say, "the yellow dock root is best to be taken when either the blood or the liver is affected by choler." This may explain its use in the past for various types of cancers. The Chinese use it for constipation, boils, and fungal infections. The leaves used to be eaten as part of a spring tonic, but research has shown them to have large quantities of oxalates, which are implicated in kidney stones and gout. The root, however, does not cause this problem in the dosages given. According to Vogel, the European version of dock was one of the few herbs adopted into Native American usage, along with the indigenous varieties. The Dakotas used the leaves as a poultice to relieve boils, while the roots were used for their tannins by the Ojibwas for closing and healing cuts.

Parts used

Root.

Active constituents

Anthraquinone glycosides, tannins, rumicin, and oxalates.

How it works in the body

It is the anthraquinones which are responsible for the laxative effect for which this herb is mainly used. They work by stimulating the colon to expel waste and toxins. In small amounts anything which has a laxative effect may be cleansing for the body, but large amounts would have a purgative effect, causing excessive peristalsis, resulting in griping pains. However, at the right dosage the plant gives a gentle action well suited to relieve moderate constipation. It also acts to aid the digestive processes. Combined with other herbs, yellow dock is well suited to assist the liver in the cleansing of toxins from the skin, and is used in complaints such as eczema, psoriasis, and acne. In the musculoskeletal system, where there is often a build-up of toxins resulting from constipation, the herb is again cleansing.

Applications

The root is made into a decoction. Take 100 ml (4 fl oz) daily for short periods for constipation. For skin problems, combine with marigold and cleavers and use 100 ml (4 fl oz) daily of the three herbs combined. As a tincture, take 2½ ml (50 drops) three times a day.

Indications

- Clears constipation and aids the digestion.
- Skin complaints such as eczema, psoriasis, and acne.
- Arthritic complaints.
- To clear fungal infections.

Contraindications

Do not take during pregnancy or while breastfeeding.

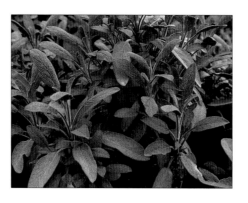

SAGE

Labiatae SALVIA OFFICINALIS

Garden, or red sage as it is also called, comes from the Mediterranean regions and is widely cultivated in many other countries throughout the world. There are many varieties, but red sage is the medicinal herb, growing to about 60 cm (2 ft) high, with paired, wrinkled, reddish-purple leaves. The flowers are also reddish purple. The leaves, when crushed, have a distinctive odor.

History

Salvia comes from the Latin *salvere*, or to be saved, which refers to the plant's long history of medicinal use. In the Middle Ages a favorite homily was *cur mariatur homo cui Salvia crescit in horto?*, meaning "Why should a man die while sage grows in his garden?" Various superstitions surround the herb, for example it is said that where sage grows prosperity in business matters follows. In France sage is a symbol used to ease grief, and is often sown in graveyards. Some varieties have been used as a substitute for tea, and on some Greek islands the leaves are made into sweets. It has also been used as snuff, and powdered to make a paste for use in whitening the teeth, similar to a toothpaste. According to Vogel, sage was used by lower California Indians, the seeds being ground and stirred in water to prevent dryness in the mouth and throat. The roots were used by the Catawbas as an ointment for sores.

Parts used

Leaves.

Active constituents

Volatile oil with thujone, cineole, borneol and camphor, diterpene bitters, flavonoids, phenolic acids (e.g., Rosmarinic), and salviatannin.

How it works in the body

It is mainly the thujone that is responsible for sage's antiseptic properties, which makes it invaluable for use as a gargle and mouthwash. It also acts as a circulatory and mild digestive stimulant. In the reproductive system, sage can be used to bring on a delayed period, and in menopause can be taken to relieve sweats and balance hormonal changes. Sage has also been an ingredient in asthma herbal cigarettes, with the rosmarinic acid acting as an anti-inflammatory and antispasmodic.

Applications

Take sage as an infusion, 200 ml (8 fl oz) a day, or use as a gargle or mouthwash, 100 ml (4 fl oz), two to three times a day. (*See* Herbal Methods, gargles and mouthwashes p.21). The tincture can be taken 2 ml (40 drops), twice a day.

Indications

- As a mouthwash, use for sore or bleeding gums and for mouth ulcers. As a gargle, use for sore throats, tonsillitis, and similar problems. Also use as a breath freshener.
- To aid circulation and stimulate digestion.
- To bring on a delayed period.
- In menopause to relieve sweats and balance hormones.

Contraindications

Do not take during pregnancy.

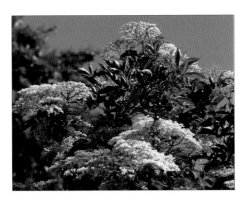

ELDERFLOWER

Caprifoliaceae SAMBUCUS NIGRA

The elder is a tree common in Europe and the British Isles. When flowering the tree is a mass of creamy-white, flat-topped blossoms, which are followed by bunches of black berries. It grows in woods and on wasteground, and is now widely found in other parts of the world.

History

The name *Sambucus* comes from the Greek for sambuke, or musical instrument, which is made from the wood of the tree; *nigra* refers to the black berries. The elder tree has possibly more folklore associated with it than almost any other plant—nearly every country has legends which include it. The Greeks and many others assigned it magic powers. The Englishman John Evelyn recommended an infusion of elderflowers in vinegar to be added to salads for medicinal benefits. The berries were also made into wine as a tonic for colds and flu, to be taken just before bedtime. The Iroquois, and also the Menominees, used the infusion of either the berries or inner bark of *Sambucus canadensis* as a treatment for fever, to induce sweating, and also as a painkiller. The Meskwakis used it to loosen phlegm.

Parts used
Flowers, berries, leaves, bark.

Active constituents
Triterpenes (including ursolic acid), fixed oils, flavonoids, phenolic acids.

How it works in the body
Generally, the herb has an anti-inflammatory action, attributed to the presence of the ursolic acid. The benefits are mostly directed at the respiratory system; it is a specific for nasal catarrh. It is also useful for allergies, such as hayfever and allergic rhinitis. The herb has a diaphoretic effect which encourages the loss of toxins through sweating, so is particularly useful in colds and flu, where it will lower a fever and reduce excess catarrh. It will in addition relieve earache where this is due to the buildup of mucous, and is also used as a gargle for sore throats. Finally, the plant works on the urinary system, having a mild diuretic effect, again encouraging the elimination of waste material, which is helpful in arthritic conditions.

Applications
Use the flowers as an infusion for colds and flu, drinking 200 ml (8 fl oz), three times a day. Use the flowers also as a tincture in allergic as well as arthritic conditions, taking 5 ml (1 tsp), three times a day. The berries can be prepared by decoction. Being rich in vitamin C, they are used for colds and flu—take 200 ml (8 fl oz) twice a day. The leaves are made into an infusion which can be used as a gargle or mouthwash, and the bark is made into a decoction for the same purpose. (Remember to only take small amounts of bark from the tree or it may be damaged beyond recovery.) Elder leaves have been used as an ointment for chilblains, wounds, and dry skin. Use an infusion of the flowers in the bath to soothe dry skin, and as an inhalant to clear blocked sinuses.

Indications
- Coughs and colds, to promote the dispersal of catarrh.
- Gargle for sore throats.
- Soothe dry skin.
- Healing agent for chilblains and wounds.
- Arthritic conditions.

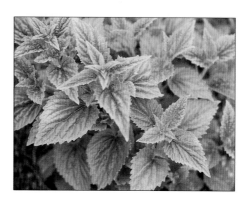

SKULLCAP
Labiatae SCUTELLARIA LATERIFLORA

Native to North America, skullcap is also found in Europe, but the variety is not thought to have the same medicinal qualities as its New World counterpart. The plant has thin, square stems, and grows to about 60 cm (2 ft). The paired leaves have fine hairs. The flowers are blue, and the seed capsules give the herb its name, being shaped like a cap. Skullcap is generally found alongside rivers and streams, and thrives in watery surroundings.

History
One of this plant's common names is mad dog skullcap, referring to its traditional use in North America for hydrophobia or rabies. It is also known as Virginian skullcap, after the state where it grows abundantly. In Native American use this herb was predominantly used for the reproductive system to relieve symptoms of premenstrual syndrome. In the 19th century, skullcap's properties and effects on the nervous system were extolled, and the plant became a cure-all for all disorders connected with this system, including hysteria, St Vitus's Dance, and epilepsy. Today's usage confirms its role in the treatment of nervous system ailments, even though skullcap is perhaps not quite the cure-all it was once thought to be.

Parts used
Whole herb.

Active constituents
Flavonoid glycoside, scutellarin, iridoids, volatile oils and waxes, tannins.

How it works in the body
Skullcap, as described above, works mainly on the nervous system. It acts as a sedative, both mentally and physically, to calm and sustain an over-excited system. It can be used where there is stress and tension present. Some species of skullcap have been found to contain constituents which have anti-inflammatory and anti-allergenic properties, and it is possible this extends to *Scutelleria laterilflora*, but further research has yet to be carried out. One species found in China has a beneficial effect in liver disorders such as hepatitis, actually improving liver-function tests. Skullcap's sedative effect also helps to alleviate period or ovarian pain.

Applications
Skullcap may be taken as an infusion, 200 ml (8 fl oz), three times a day. The tincture is taken 2 ml (40 drops), three times a day.

Indications
- In conditions of stress and anxiety.
- Included with other herbs such as lavender and passion flower in a remedy for insomnia.
- Ovarian and period pain.

Benefits of skullcap

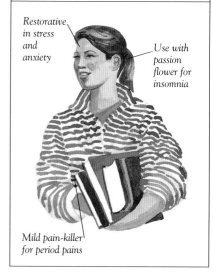

Restorative in stress and anxiety

Use with passion flower for insomnia

Mild pain-killer for period pains

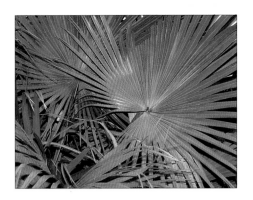

SAW PALMETTO

Palmaceae SERENOA SERRULATA SABAL SERRULATA

This plant originates from North America, more particularly from the Atlantic Coast, including South Carolina, Florida, and southern California. It is a palm which grows to about three meters (9 ft), with large fanned-out leaves. The flowers are pale, and the fruit a deep reddish-brown.

History

The Native Americans have a long history of usage of this and related species for medicinal purposes, while the Mayas used *Sabal japa* extensively. The inner bark was made into a decoction and then used to treat dysentery, abdominal pains, and snake and insect bites. In addition, a poultice of the bark was used topically for ulcers. The Houma Indians apparently drank the decoction for kidney problems, while the dried root was used for high blood pressure. Vogel lists sources which tell of early settlers using the palm branches to make brooms. Some early settlers apparently saw animals thriving on a diet of the berries and added them to their medicinal stores. Further research is needed into the extensive properties of this plant.

Parts used

Berries.

Active constituents

Essential oil, fixed oil, sterols, polysaccharides.

How it works in the body

As the early settlers discovered, saw palmetto is a tonic which builds and restores body tissue. The sterols have an anabolic action, which helps to build and maintain weight, so can usefully be given to those who are convalescing or have lost weight through illness or debility. In the reproductive system it has useful applications for both men and women. In men it is given to enhance the sex drive and to treat impotence and infertility. In women it is thought to have an estrogenic action and can be used where this is a cause of disorder in the reproductive system. As a urinary tract tonic it is used where there is weakness in the neck of the bladder, and also as a diuretic to improve urinary flow. Saw palmetto has been shown to be effective in treating enlargement of the prostate in men.

Applications

The infusion may be taken 100 ml (4 fl oz), twice daily. The tincture may be taken 2 ml (40 drops), three times a day.

Indications

- In convalescence or debility to restore weight and improve vitality.
- For men, to enhance the sex drive and to treat impotence and infertility.
- For women, to restore estrogenic levels.
- As a diuretic to improve urinary flow.
- For enlargement of the prostate.

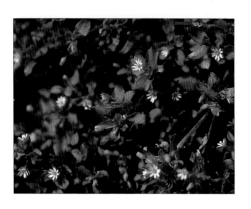

CHICKWEED

Caryophyllaceae STELLARIA MEDIA

Chickweed is a common garden weed originating in Europe, which now grows extensively worldwide. The plant grows close to the ground, with dark-green, oval leaves and has tiny, white, star-like flowers, which give it its name.

History

As a food the leaves have been used fresh in salads, and as a source of vitamin C—at one time it was recommended for use against scurvy. When boiled as a vegetable, it resembled spinach in taste and texture, and was often added to soups. Chickweed had a reputation for aiding weight loss, possibly due to its property as a lymph cleanser, In addition, it was once used as a treatment for hydrophobia! The plant has been highly thought of by herbalists through the ages, from Gerard and Culpeper, to the present time.

Parts used

The leaves and flowers together.

Active constituents

Saponin glycosides, coumarins, flavonoids, carboxylic acids, triterpenoids, and vitamin C.

How it works in the body

Internally, it is thought the saponins are responsible for the relief of itching. It is particularly noted for its cooling qualities, and is especially soothing when applied to skin problems presenting as hot and itchy. It is thought to be useful on wounds to reduce scarring. Additionally, the combined constituents are thought to be beneficial for arthritic conditions, while topically the whole plant has a soothing, healing quality. The herb works also on the digestive system in small amounts, soothing and healing the digestive tract.

Applications

As an infusion, internally, take 200 ml (8 fl oz) twice a day. Externally, the infusion can be used in the bath to reduce inflammation. Also, use as a cream or ointment twice a day for skin complaints, or as a poultice if required. Note: It is thought that the fresh herb is better used for creams, ointments, and poultices rather than the dried variety. The cream is best kept in the refrigerator, which will enhance its cooling qualities. As a tincture, use internally 1 ml (20 drops) three times a day.

Indications

- Internally for eczema, psoriasis, and related irritative skin complaints.
- Externally as a cream or ointment to reduce scarring on new wounds.
- As a poultice for boils and abscesses.
- Internally for arthritis complaints, where there is pain and stiffness.
- As a tea for sore throats and coughs, generally healing and cleansing to the lungs.
- For the digestive system to gently encourage calming and healing of the gut.

Contraindications

This herb may have a laxative effect in large doses. **Avoid** during pregnancy.

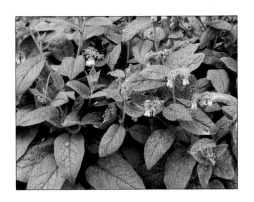

COMFREY

Boraginaceae SYMPHYTUM OFFICINALE

The main feature of this plant are the leaves. The plant itself grows to about one meter (3 ft) high and the leaves are large, oval, and bristly. The flowers are drooping and bell-like, either white or purple. Originating from Europe and parts of Asia, this herb is particularly common where there is marshy or watery ground. Today it is also found in North America and Australia.

History

The name Comfrey comes from *con firma*, which means to "join bones," while its botanical name *Symphytum* comes from the Greek meaning to "unite bones."

Parts used

Leaf, internally. Root, externally.

Active constituents

Allantoin, pyrrolizidine alkaloids, phenolic acids including rosmarinic, mucilage, volatile oil, tannins, and saponins.

How it works in the body

The principal ingredient allantoin works to promote the healing of tissues within the body. It is complemented by the rosmarinic acid, an anti-inflammatory agent. The mucilage is demulcent and works to soothe irritative conditions, both internally and externally. The tannins act as an astringent. The pyrrolizidine alkaloids are thought to be damaging to the liver. These pyrrolizidine alkaloids are mainly concentrated in the root of the plant, and therefore there is common agreement by the main bodies of herbal practitioners that this should not be taken internally. It has, however, also been substantiated that the leaf does not present this problem, and may be taken internally under the guidance of a qualified herbal or medical practitioner. Both the leaf and the root can be safely used externally.

Applications

The leaf may be made as a tincture, and used under the direction of a herbal or medical practitioner for the purpose of healing stomach ulcers and other disorders, and in the respiratory system for conditions such as bronchitis. The leaf may also be made as a poultice or compress, and applied to sprains or bruised areas. It is also possible to make an infused oil from the leaf, which may be applied to the skin over an area where fractures or a break in the bone has occurred, and to scar tissue. Comfrey infused oil can be used as a massage oil to relieve stiff and aching joints in arthritic conditions. Comfrey ointment may be used instead of the oil in all cases mentioned.

Indications

- The tincture under supervision for stomach ulcers and irritable bowel syndrome, and also for bronchitic conditions.
- The oil or ointment for all cases of injury, sprains, breaks, and bruises.
- The oil may be rubbed in in cases of arthritic joints.
- The oil on scar tissue to aid healing.

Contraindications

Never take the leaf internally without the supervision of a qualified herbal or medical practitioner. Never apply any comfrey preparations to an open wound, cut, or graze. **Never** take the root internally.

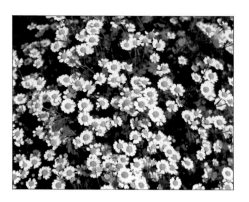

FEVERFEW

Compositae TANACETUM PARTHENIUM

This plant is native in southern Europe, but has spread widely to many parts of the world, including North America. It grows to about 60 cm (2 ft) and is daisy-like in appearance, with yellow central florets surrounded by an outer ring of white ray florets. It differs from other camomiles in that the central disk is nearly flat rather than conical. The leaves are alternate, yellowish-green, and fern-like.

History

Feverfew is a corruption of *febrifuge*, which means to bring down a fever. *Parthenium* derives from the Greek *pyrethrum*, or fire, which some say refers to the hotness of the root, while others say alludes to the heat or burning associated with a fever. Traditionally, it was planted in gardens surrounding dwellings to purify the air and ward off disease. This may be due in part to its reputation as an insect repellent. The tincture was used as a wash to alleviate the pain of insect bites and stings, and, if applied to exposed skin, the diluted tincture was said to act as an effective insect repellent.

Parts used

Leaves.

Active constituents

Volatile oil containing spiroketal enol ethers; sesquiterpene lactones including parthenolide; acetylene derivatives, mainly in the root.

How it works in the body

Feverfew's action against fevers is thought to be due to the sesquiterpene lactones, which inhibit the release of arachidonic acid in the body. These ingredients have also been shown to inhibit other substances which contribute to anti-blood clotting. In the reproductive system, feverfew has an age-old function of promoting menstrual flow. Its main use today is to prevent and alleviate headaches, especially migraine. It is thought from research that the sesquiterpene lactones, among the other constituents, inhibit the secretion of serotonin, which is implicated in the onset of migraine. Another area of research is looking at the role feverfew has in the musculo-skeletal system, where its inhibitory effects are thought to help control pain in conditions such as arthritis.

Applications

The fresh leaf is taken as a preventative. Two leaves daily may be taken, wrapped in a piece of bread. The tincture may be taken, ½ ml (10 drops), once a day. Tablets and capsules are available commercially.

Indications

- To reduce fevers.
- To promote menstrual flow.
- To prevent and also to alleviate headaches, especially migraine.
- A pain killer, with other herbs, in arthritic conditions.

Contraindications

Do not take in pregnancy. **Do not** take this herb if you are receiving medication such as Warfarin which thins the blood. The fresh leaf should only be taken with bread or similar substances as it may cause ulcers if it comes into contact with the mucous membranes present in the mouth.

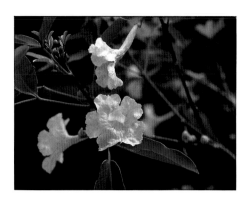

PAO D'ARCO

Bignoniaceae TABEBUIA SPECIES

There are many different species of Pao d'Arco (its Portuguese name) or lapacho (its Spanish name). It is a tree which originates from Brazil, but has spread to other countries in South America and in North America. The tree grows to about 30 meters (100 ft), and has pinkish-purple flowers.

History

One of the many varieties of Pao d'Arco is often grown as an ornamental garden tree in North America. It is also commonly known as taheebo. The varieties are difficult to distinguish and there is dispute as to which varieties have the specified medicinal qualities. *Tabebuia avellanedae* and *Tabebuia impetignosa* are the most commonly used medicinally. Pao d'Arco has been used for over a thousand years for its curative value.

Parts used

Inner bark.

Active constituents

The main active ingredient in this plant is the quinones, of which there are 18, the main ones being naphthoquinones, of which lapa-

chol and a form of lapachone are some of the most important. The bioflavonoid quercetin, lapachenole, carnosol, indoles, coenzyme Q, alkaloids, and steroidal saponins.

How it works in the body

Lapachol was isolated as early as 1882, and in 1956 its antibacterial action was confirmed by research in Brazil which makes Pao d'Arco a valuable natural antibiotic. Further tests showed derivatives of this constituent also had antifungal properties effective against ringworm, vaginal thrush, and gastrointestinal candidiasis. Carnosol is a strong antioxidant which mops up free radicals in the body, and is thought to be responsible for the reputation of Pao d'Arco as an anticarcinogenic. In addition, the indoles have been identified as being active in detoxifying the body from carcinogens. A form of lapachone has an antiviral action which has been used against viruses such as herpes simplex and polio, but has also been used against retroviruses which are particularly implicated in cancer, especially leukemia, and AIDS. Pao d'Arco also demonstrates activity against

some tropical parasites, and the alkaloids show some evidence of benefit in diabetes. Its detoxifying element is used in skin complaints, and its anti-inflammatory action for conditions such as cystitis, prostatitis, and intestinal inflammation.

Applications

As a decoction, drink 200 ml (8 fl oz), three times a day. As a tincture take 3 ml (60 drops) three times a day. For vaginal thrush, soak a tampon in a strong infusion of the herb and insert as usual, in addition to taking the herb orally. Tablets are available commercially.

Indications

- Bacterial and viral infection, especially ear, nose, and throat.
- Fungal problems, including vaginal thrush and candidiasis of the gastrointestinal tract.
- Cancer and leukemia, in addition to orthodox treatments.
- Inflammatory conditions, including cystitis, prostatitis, and stomach inflammation.
- HIV, AIDS, chronic fatigue syndrome, and other immune-related illnesses.
- Flu and colds.

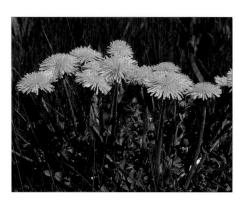

DANDELION

Compositae TARAXACUM OFFICINALE (*pu gong ying*)

Chinese pharmaceutical name: *herba taraxaci mongolici cum radice*

The shiny leaves are noted for their jagged, tooth-like shape. The flowers are bright yellow. This well-known weed grows on wasteland and cultivated areas alike. Originating in Europe and Asia, it now grows in many countries.

History

The name comes from the Greek *taraxos*, or "disorder", and *aka*, or "remedy."

Parts used

Leaves and root.

Active constituents

Sesquiterpene lactones, triterpenes, phenolic acids, polysaccharides, carotenoids, and vitamins A and C, potassium.

How it works in the body

The leaves contain a high amount of potassium, which balances their function as a powerful diuretic. This is in contrast to orthodox diuretics, which need a potassium supplement to balance the requirements of the body. In Chinese terms this herb resolves painful urinary ailments. The root functions differently, being used to treat the liver to improve its function, and as a mild laxative. In Chinese usage, dandelion is indicated for heat disorders, especially in the liver, where there are red, swollen, and painful eyes, and for damp-heat jaundice. Both leaf and root act as a tonic to the gallbladder. Its detoxifying properties are thought to have a beneficial effect on removing the effects of pollution on the body . In addition, the Chinese use it where there are firm or hard abscesses, especially involving the breast and digestive system. For these it can be used internally and topically. In women who are breastfeeding, it is used to promote lactation. The Chinese properties are those of bitter, sweet, and cold.

Applications

Use fresh in salads or soups. Include in tonic wines to cleanse the system and eliminate toxins. Take one sherryglassful a day. Use the leaf as an infusion, taking 200 ml (8 fl oz) three times daily for water retention. Also use the leaf as a tincture, 2 ml (40 drops) three times a day. The root is prepared as a decoction. Take 200 ml (8 fl oz) twice a day. As a tincture the root can be taken 2 ml (40 drops), three times a day. The Chinese dosage is 9–30 g (½–1½ oz).

Indications

- **The leaf** in cases of water retention, e.g., in high blood pressure. Also to promote removal of waste products from the kidneys, e.g., in arthritic conditions.
- **The root** as a tonic to the liver, especially in arthritic conditions to improve removal of toxins, and in skin conditions such as eczema, psoriasis, and acne. Also as a gentle laxative. Taken before a meal, the root has a bitter action which helps to promote appetite.
- **The leaf and root** as a gallbladder tonic, especially where there are gallstones.
- As a detoxifier where there has been undue strain on the body, e.g., excess alcohol consumption.

Contraindications

As the bitter effect has a stimulating action on the digestion, take this remedy after meals where there is excess acid, or stomach ulcers. The Chinese caution that overdosage can cause mild diarrhea.

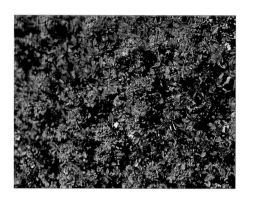

THYME
Labiatae THYMUS VULGARIS

Common or garden thyme is a native of the Mediterranean, and cultivated in many parts of the world. Wild thyme is native to Britain and Europe. There are a huge number of varieties of thyme, the wild thyme often being used similarly to common thyme. It is a shrub growing to around 30 cm (2 ft), with pinkish-purple flowers.

History
Thymus probably comes from a Greek word meaning to fumigate, probably due to its use as an incense and as an antiseptic, but it is also suggested it comes from the Greek *thumus*, meaning courage. In England it was embroidered on tokens given to knights to enhance their valor in battle. It was also used by the Romans to give flavor to cheese and to liqueurs. The honey from bees fed on thyme has been highly praised. It is, of course, also used to flavor cooking today. Culpeper said of thyme that it was, "a noble strengthener of the lungs, as notable a one as grows, neither is there scarce a better remedy growing for that disease in children which they commonly called the chin-cough (whooping cough)."

Parts used
Whole herb, essential oil.

Active constituents
Volatile oil especially thymol with cineole, borneol and others, flavonoids, caffeic acid, tannins.

How it works in the body
As Culpeper suggested, thyme is primarily a remedy for the respiratory system. It is the thymol which is responsible for its expectorant and antiseptic qualities, and this is invaluable for chest infections and other respiratory ailments. However, the thymol is also useful in the urinary tract system, where it is beneficial as an antiseptic. The thymol, together with other constituents, act together as an antispasmodic, and this has a sedative effect which is used particularly in children's asthma and for those who suffer from hayfever. In addition, there is an antilarval action. In the muscoloskeletal system, the oil can be used topically in a base oil as a counterirritant, that is, to draw blood to an area and to warm a cold joint in cases of rheumatic disorder.

Applications
As an infusion, take 200 ml (8 fl oz), twice a day. As tincture, take 2 ml (40 drops), three times daily. As a syrup, thyme can be combined with licorice and taken for coughs and sore throats, 10 ml (2 tsp), three times a day. The essential oil may be combined with others in a base oil, or on its own, 2 drops in 50 ml (4 tbsp) base oil as a rub to stimulate circulation to warm cold joints. The essential oil may also be used when added to water as an inhalation to ease tight airways. Add the infusion to the bath to relax tired and aching muscles.

Indications
- Respiratory complaints, such as asthma, bronchitis, hayfever, sore throats, and coughs.
- Arthritic complaints where there are cold joints.
- Tired and aching muscles.
- Urinary tract infections (in combination with other herbs).
- Worms.

Contraindications
Do not take more than the stated dosage. **Do not** take the essential oil internally. The oil should **not** be used externally during pregnancy.

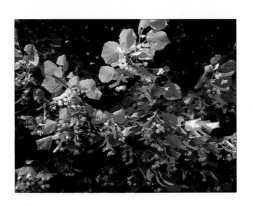

LIMEBLOSSOM

Tiliaceae TILIA EUROPAEA

Limeblossom, or limeflower as it is also known, is a tree that grows to a height of 30 meters (100 ft) with heart-shaped leaves and yellowish-white flowers which hang in clusters. It originates from Europe, although there is a species which also grows in North America, *Tilia americana*, which has similar properties.

History

The wood is much used in carving, being light in color and easy to work. The honey from the flowers is regarded as one of the most delicately flavored in the world. In many of the old herbals, the use of limeblossoms were said to have a sedative, antispasmodic effect in cases of epilepsy, and it was thought that if a patient was taken to lie under the tree, it would help to reduce the severity of a seizure. Quite often the tree is found along streets, and is blamed for a sticky, black substance which drops on to parked cars. In fact, this is due to a parasite which lives on the tree, rather than the tree itself. The North American variety, which has the common name basswood, was used, according to Vogel, by Forest Indians for the treatment of burns.

Parts used

Flowers.

Active constituents

Volatile oil, flavonoids, mucilage, phenolic acids, tannins.

How it works in the body

The relaxing qualities of limeblossom make it extremely useful in the nervous system, where it has applications for conditions requiring an antispasmodic action, for example, in cases of stress and tension. It is helpful as a remedy for sleeplessness due to its sedative action. For headaches, especially caused by excess catarrh, this is an excellent remedy. In the cardiovascular system, limeblossom is used to treat high blood pressure, and has a reputation for helping to lower cholesterol associated with arteriosclerosis. In the digestive system, it is useful for indigestion associated with nervous tension. It has a diaphoretic action, which helps the body to sweat out toxins. This, combined with its anti-catarrhal properties, makes it helpful in colds and flu.

Applications

As an infusion, use 200 ml (8 fl oz) three times a day for indigestion, stress, headaches, and general tension. Use the infusion in the bath to calm and relax. Take the tincture between 2½–5 ml (½–1 tsp) at bedtime for sleeplessness. Take 2 ml (40 drops) three times a day for high blood pressure.

Indications

- Indigestion and stress-related stomach complaints.
- Insomnia.
- Headaches, especially where there is excess catarrh.
- Symptoms of colds and flu.
- High blood pressure, to lower cholesterol levels.

Contraindications

Do not use this herb in low blood pressure.

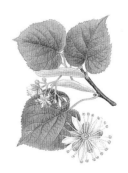

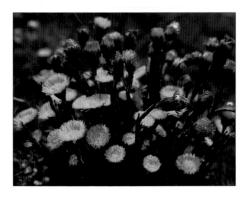

COLTSFOOT

Compositae TUSSILAGO FARFARA *(kuan dong hua)*

The plant has a flowering stem with star-like, yellow flowers and broad green leaves. It originated in Europe and Asia and now grows extensively in North America.

History

The plant's botanical name *Tussilago farfara* indicates its usage, *tussive* meaning cough and *farfara*, to go. In other words, dispels coughs. Another name was *Filius ante patrem* or "the son before the father," as the flowers appear first, then die off before the leaves grow. The herb has long been used as a symbol of herbal medicine and enjoys an old reputation as a remedy for lung problems, including asthma and bronchitis, being included in a mixture of herbs, which was smoked. Sticks of coltsfoot rock are still sold for the relief of coughs. In China the flowers are preferred, while in Europe the leaves are used exclusively since it is thought there is a higher proportion of toxic constituents in the flowers.

Parts used

Leaves.

Active constituents

Flavonoids, mucilage (about 8 per cent, consisting mainly of polysaccharides), pyrrolizidine alkaloids, tannin.

How it works in the body

The flavonoids have an antispasmodic and anti-inflammatory effect which eases spasm in the lungs during asthma and bronchitis attacks, allowing easier breathing. The polysaccharides are anti-inflammatory, which helps to calm irritated lung tissue. They also act as an expectorant for excess phlegm and mucous. Together these constituents work to improve the immune system and promote a healthy respiratory system. The pyrrolizidine alkaloids are thought to be harmful to the liver, but to a large extent are destroyed when prepared as a decoction.

Applications

The herb is prepared as a decoction for the treatment of coughs and other chest complaints. It is combined with other herbs as a tobacco in herbal cigarettes to relieve the spasm in asthma and bronchitis. As a tincture take 1 ml (20 drops) twice daily to improve the lungs. It is particularly good for coughs when used as a syrup. The Chinese dosage is 1.5–9 g (1⁄16–1⁄2 oz).

Indications

- Dry and irritating coughs.
- To generally improve the health of the lungs where there are lung complaints, such as asthma or bronchitis.

Contraindications

Do not use for longer than one month at a time. Only use the leaves, not the flowers. **Do not** take while pregnant or during breast-feeding. **Do not** give to children under six years old.

Benefits of coltsfoot

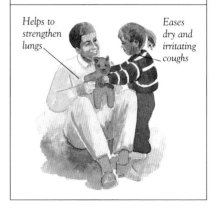

Helps to strengthen lungs

Eases dry and irritating coughs

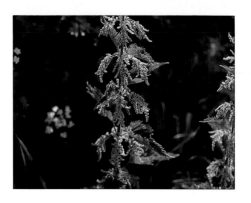

NETTLE

Urticaceae URTICA DIOICA

A plant that is familiar on wasteground. Found in many parts of the world, it grows to about 1½ meters (4½ ft) with serrated green leaves, the flowers in clusters. Sometimes the male and female flowers are found on the same plant, but more usually they are on separate plants. The main feature of the nettle is its covering of fine hairs, swollen at the base, from which arises its stinging effect.

History

The plant's name arises from the Latin *uro*, or "I burn," referring to the stinging qualities of the plant, and *dioica*, or, two houses, which refers to the male and female plants being separate. The common name of nettle is from the Anglo-Saxon and comes from the word *noedl* or needle. The stinging nettle was said to have been introduced to Britain by the Romans, who rubbed it on their joints, the stinging encouraging blood to the area, helping to offset the effects of Britain's damp, cold climate. It has been used for many purposes, for example the tough fibers to weave cloth. This was immortalized in Hans Christian Andersen's story of the princess and the eleven swans: the cloaks she had to make for them by sunrise were of nettle, and when the sun's rays touched them, the youngest of the brothers was left with one arm as a swan's wing. It has also been used to make paper. In 1835, after visiting Native Americans and taking their advice, Vogel, a doctor in British Columbia found that nettle cured his patients' scurvy.

Parts used

Herb and root.

Active constituents

Chlorophyll, indoles (e.g., histamine and serotonin), acetylcholine, vitamin C, iron, and dietary fiber.

How it works in the body

Although the growing nettle stings externally, it has no such effect when it has been subjected to heat, either in cooking or when made into an infusion. Ironically, it is used in skin complaints as an anti-allergenic, and can be used to treat eczema and related allergies when taken internally. It is also anti-hemorrhagic, and can be used as an astringent to stop excessive bleeding, either from wounds, or in the reproductive system to diminish heavy bleeding. The iron and vitamin C content make it an excellent tonic for anemia and lack of iron. It was used, along with the other first herbs of spring, as a spring tonic. The root has been used to treat enlarged prostate.

Applications

As an infusion, take 200 ml (8 fl oz), twice daily. The decoction of the roots, 200 ml (8 fl oz) daily. Tincture, take 3 ml (60 drops) three times a day. The young tops of the leaves, picked in spring, can be made into a soup which can be used daily as a tonic.

Indications

- Skin conditions, such as eczema.
- Allergic conditions, including hayfever and asthma.
- Iron tonic.
- In the reproductive system to ease heavy bleeding.
- Enlargement of the prostate (root).

Contraindications

A small number of people find that irritation occurs. If this happens, discontinue use.

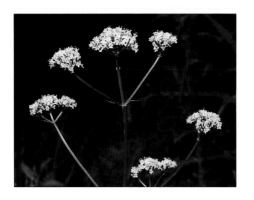

VALERIAN

Valerianaceae VALERIANA OFFICINALIS

This plant is native in Europe and Asia, and has been naturalized in North America. It grows to about 1 meter (3 ft) high. It flourishes in wet and marshy conditions, and is often found near rivers. The leaves occur in pairs and the flowers are pale pink or white, with a distinctive smell.

History

Dioscorides and Galen named this plant *phu*, which is a reference to its unpleasant odor. It is this very feature which is thought to make the plant so attractive to both rats and cats: it is suggested that the Pied Piper of Hamlyn had a supply of the herb in his pockets with which he lured the rats out of the town. In Medieval England it was employed as a remedy for epilepsy, and was given the name of "all heal." The name is thought to come from the Latin *valere*, or health. It is listed in Anglo-Saxon times as a herbal remedy. It has traditionally been used in the nervous system where there is over-stimulation. During the Second World War it was used in England for shellshock. According to Vogel, it was used as an ointment for massage, together with sea algae, by the ancient Incas.

Parts used

Root.

Active constituents

Volatile oil containing valerenic acid, iridoids known as valepotriates, alkaloids, flavonoids, sterols, and tannins.

How it works in the body

Valerian's usefulness in the nervous system is mainly due to the valepotriates, which have a sedative effect on the mind. One of its main uses is in insomnia, where it both helps the sufferer to fall asleep more quickly and allows them to wake in the morning without feeling stupefied. It is particularly useful for those whose minds are so active they cannot switch off enough to relax. It is helpful for all types of stress-related anxiety as it does not impair the ability to concentrate, but has a calming effect. It is used to treat numerous ailments, for example digestive complaints where there is a contributing stress or tension factor. It is also a muscle relaxant, and is used with other herbs in the cardiovascular system to treat high blood pressure.

Applications

As a decoction, take 100 ml (4 fl oz), twice daily. For insomnia take 200 ml (8 fl oz) at night. The tincture may be taken 2 ml (40 drops), three times a day. Tablets are available commercially.

Indications

- Insomnia, especially where there is overactivity of the mind.
- Stress and anxiety for short periods.
- Digestive complaints where stress is a factor, in combination with other herbs.
- High blood pressure, in combination with other herbs.

Contraindications

Rarely, a few people find this herb more stimulating than relaxing. If this occurs, discontinue use.

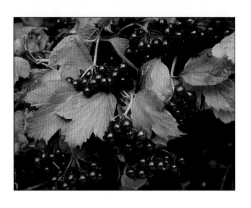

CRAMPBARK

Caprifoliaceae VIBURNUM OPULUS/PRUNIFOLIUM

Crampbark, or guelder rose as it is sometimes known, originates from both North America and Europe. It is a shrub which grows to approximately three meters (9 ft) and belongs to the same family as the elder tree. It is commonly found in woods and hedges.

History

The name guelder rose comes from a province in Holland where the plant was first cultivated. As a spasmolytic, the *opulus* variety acts on the body tissues as a whole, while the *prunifolium* is more specific in its action on the uterus. Native Americans, including the Ojibwas and Meskwakis, traditionally used the remedy for cramping conditions. The plant has been included in the US National Formulary as an antispasmodic and sedative, and for treatment of asthma.

Parts used

Bark from branches—only small amounts may be harvested at any one time as the removal of large amounts of bark may kill the tree.

Active constituents

Hydroquinones, coumarins, tannins.

How it works in the body

Crampbark acts as a muscle relaxant, particularly of smooth muscle. As mentioned, the *opulus* variety is thought to act on the body as a whole, while the *prunifolium* variety acts particularly to relax the muscles of the uterus. For this reason its main function has to do with the reproductive system, for example, to relieve the cramping which occurs during a period. It is also used in cases of threatened miscarriage, but should only be used in this context under the supervision of a qualified herbal or medical practitioner. It also has uses in many other systems of the body: in the stomach to relieve symptoms in conditions such as irritable bowel syndrome; in the respiratory system to help relax the airways in asthma; and for the musculoskeletal system to relieve the tension of arthritic pain. It is also employed in the cardiovascular system, together with other herbs to help reduce high blood pressure.

Applications

For internal use as a decoction, the herb is taken when spasm is present, rather than on a continuous basis. To relieve cramp from period or other sources, take 100 ml (4 fl oz) up to a maximum amount of six times daily. The tincture can be similarly used: take 2½ ml (50 drops) up to six times in one day. For external relief of muscle spasm, add 2 ml (40 drops) of the tincture to 30 g (1½ oz) cream, e.g. comfrey, and mix well in. It is possible to add 2 ml (40 drops) of lobelia tincture, which will enhance the antispasmodic effect. Apply up to three times a day.

Indications

- Relief of uterine and ovarian pain and cramping.
- In cases of threatened miscarriage, under the supervision of a herbal or medical practitioner only.
- Cramping of the muscles due to arthritic conditions.
- Muscle tension and spasm due to stress or night cramps.
- High blood pressure
- Asthma

Contraindications

Do not take this remedy during pregnancy. Do not take when low blood pressure is present.

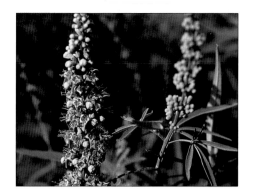

CHASTE BERRY

Verbenaceae VITEX AGNUS CASTUS

Chaste berry is a native of the Mediterranean regions. It is a shrub which grows to about seven meters (20 ft). The leaves have five to seven leaflets, dark-green on top and gray beneath, with small purple flowers and an aromatic fragrance, which give way to dark-purple berries.

History

Chaste berry has a long history as a promoter of chastity. In ceremonial rites connected with Ceres, Athenian women were said to string their couches with it. As part of a trio comprising Juno (queen of heaven) and Persephone (queen of the underworld), Ceres was queen of the earth and had two main functions: that of lawgiver and that of the source or withholder of life. Farmers held rites to her to ensure bountiful crops. This complements the age-old usage of the herb to promote fertility in women while lowering the libido of men. It is ceremonially cast in the path of male novices in Italy when they first enter monasteries, hence its common name of chaste berry, or monk's pepper. It has also been used for the relief of paralysis, general weakness, and pain in the limbs.

Parts used

Berries.

Active constituents

Iridoid glycosides (including aucibin and agnoside), volatile oil (cineol), fixed oils, alkaloids (viticine), and flavonoids (casticin).

How it works in the body

Chaste berry has distinct actions, depending on whether it is given to men or women. Commonly used as a woman's herb, it affects the pituitary gland, which sends chemical messages to regulate the hormone balance in the body. It is thought to regulate the two main hormones, estrogen and progesterone. It is invaluable in treating many disorders in the reproductive system which are due to an imbalance of these hormones, for example, PMS, irregular periods, and infertility. It can also be used to treat acne, which is a result of hormonal imbalance at puberty or menopause. For men, the herb acts to depress the male androgen hormones, which are responsible for, among other things, the male sex drive. For this reason the herb is only rarely given to men.

Applications

The tincture should be taken first thing in the morning, 1 ml (20 drops) increasing to 2 ml (40 drops) if needed, in water, daily. Tablets are available commercially. To achieve the full benefit from this remedy, it should be taken for at least three months.

Indications

- For conditions where there is hormonal imbalance.
- PMS (mood swings, bloating, breast tenderness.)
- Irregular periods.
- Migraine associated with the menstrual cycle.
- Acne, when associated with the menstrual cycle.
- Acne associated with puberty or the menopause.
- Infertility.

Contraindications

Do not exceed the stated dosage. This herb has been shown to work at these levels, and increasing the amounts taken is not advisable. If in any doubt, consult a qualified herbal practitioner.

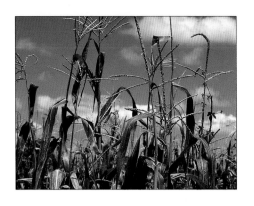

MAIZE (CORNSILK)

Gramineae ZEA MAYS *(yu mi xu)*

Originating in South America, this plant now grows in warmer climates throughout the world. It is a grass which grows to about three meters (10 ft). The cornsilk refers to the fronds around the corn cob, and once the female flower has been fertilized these turn brown and the yellow kernels grow.

History

Maize is primarily a foodstuff so the medicinal part—the fronds or "silks"—is usually discarded. Maize has long been used medicinally by Native Americans, usually as a poultice for skin conditions. It was quickly adopted by pioneers as a useful diuretic and remedy for cystitis. Chinese research has found evidence of its usefulness in the circulatory system, mainly as an agent to lower blood pressure and to reduce blood-clotting time.

Parts used

Cornmeal (kernels) externally, cornsilk internally.

Active constituents

Saponins, allantoin, sterols, alkaloid (hordenine), mucilage, vitamins C and K, and potassium.

How it works in the body

This herb works mainly in the urinary tract. The saponins largely act as an anti-inflammatory in the body and the allantoin as a healing agent, with the mucilage giving a demulcent or soothing effect to irritated tissues. The potassium balances out the diuretic effect of the herb, which is used in conditions of water retention. Their combined action is useful for a number of urinary tract conditions, such as cystitis and prostatitis. Vitamin K is a fat soluble vitamin that is essential for blood clotting within the body.

Applications

Use cornsilk as an infusion, fresh or dried. In urinary tract infections, take 1 cup, 200 ml (8 fl oz) three times a day. Use a decoction of the meal as a poultice for wounds and sores. As a tincture take 3 ml (50 drops) three times a day for conditions such as cystitis. The Chinese dosage is 15–30 g (¾–1½ oz).

Indications

- To reduce water retention, for example in high blood pressure.
- Frequent urination, e.g. cystitis.
- Difficulty in passing water, e.g. prostatitis.
- For kidney problems, e.g., kidney stones.

Contraindications

Do not take in conditions of low blood pressure.

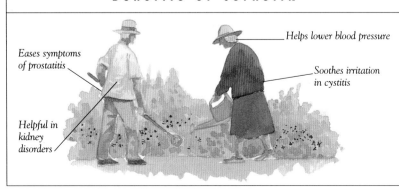

Benefits of cornsilk

Eases symptoms of prostatitis

Helpful in kidney disorders

Helps lower blood pressure

Soothes irritation in cystitis

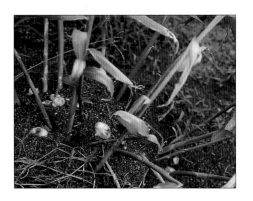

GINGER

Zingiberaceae ZINGIBER OFFICINALE *(sheng jiang)*

Originally from Asia, ginger is now also grown in many countries, including China, North America, Jamaica, Africa, and in other tropical countries. The aerial part of the plant consists of a green stalk with narrow leaves and a spike of yellow or white flowers. It is the root or rhizome which has the long, tuberous joints familiar in cooking. The plant needs to be a year old before use can be made of the root. Research continues into the benefits of ginger, with recent studies confirming its use as an antiemetic, and also as valuable in the treatment of bacillary dysentry.

History

Said to be used since Greek and Roman times for its medicinal benefits as well as culinary use, the Romans introduced this plant to Britain.

Parts used

Root or rhizome.

Active constituents

Volatile oil, phenolic compounds, including gingerols and shogaols.

How it works in the body

The phenolic compounds are the agents responsible for relaxing the muscles of the stomach, and this may also explain their effect in easing travel or motion sickness. Fresh or dried, the root has been shown to minimize vomiting. In addition, the phenolic ingredients act within the stomach as a sedative and painkiller, which helps to reduce over-activity of the gut. In stomach infections, the oil acts as an antiseptic and an anti-inflammatory. The gingerols alone are thought to be responsible for ginger's action as a liver protective. In the cardiovascular system, ginger is thought to also reduce cholesterol levels, while at the same time increasing a sluggish circulation. In China, the fresh rhizome is used to warm the stomach to ease vomiting, and to fight off colds, chills and coughs, especially where there is phlegm, and for bloating, while the dried rhizome is used for abdominal pain. The Chinese properties are those of acrid and warm.

Applications

Take ginger as an infusion, 200 ml (8 fl oz) three times a day for digestion or for nausea. For travel sickness, combine with camomile in a flask and take before and during a journey. The tincture may be taken 1 ml (20 drops) three times a day to improve the circulation, and for coughs, colds, and flu symptoms. The Chinese dosage indicates 3–9 g (⅛–½ oz).

Indications

• Travel and motion sickness.
• Indigestion and nausea; sickness in pregnancy.
• Sluggish circulation, especially where there are cold hands and feet.
• High cholesterol.
• Colds, flu, and coughs.
• Over-activity of the gut, wind, and bloating.

Contraindications

In Chinese terms, this herb should not be used in cases of lung heat, or stomach heat with vomiting. It should be used with caution in lung infections with fevers, or with irritative digestive complaints, such as ulcers and acid indigestion.

ADDITIONAL HERBS

A brief description of herbs used or mentioned in the book but not listed in

the Herbal Directory.

Agrimony
Agrimonia eupatoria Astringent and tonic properties, making it a valuable remedy for the treatment of childhood diarrhea and urinary incontinence.

Arnica
Arnica montana One of the best herbs for healing bruising and sprains. **Caution**: *Never take internally.* Should not be used if the skin is broken.

Bladderwrack
Fucus vesiculosus Very useful in regulating the thyroid. Helps an under-active thyroid and goiter.

Boneset
Eupatorium perfoliatum One of the best remedies for the relief of symptoms associated with flu—relieves fevers, catarrh, aches, and pains.

Borage
Borago officinalis Benefits the adrenal glands, helping to restore function after the use of steroids. Also helps boost the immune system.

Bugleweed
Lycopus europaens Specific use for over-active thyroid, helping with symptoms of palpitations, shaking, and breathing difficulties.

Catnip
Nepeta cataria Traditionally used for the treatment of colds and flu, but also relaxing and calming properties. Especially suitable for children with fevers.

Cayenne
Capsicum minimum Stimulant and tonic, helping digestive and circulatory disorders. Use in small amounts—approximately one-quarter of recommended general dosage.

Celery seed
Apium graveolens Antiseptic useful in treatment of urinary problems, and also, with dandelion leaf, in rheumatic conditions.

Cinnamon
Cinnamomum zeylanicum Helps to relieve nausea and vomiting, and mild cases of diarrhea.

Cloves
Eugenia caryophyllus Stimulant to the digestive system. Powerful local antiseptic and mild anesthetic, can also be used for toothache. **Caution:** *Do not swallow the clove pieces.*

Damiana
Turnera aphrodisiaca Helps strengthen the nervous system, and useful as anti-depressant. Strengthens the male reproductive system, thus enhancing libido.

Elecampane
Inula helenium Helpful for irritating bronchial coughs, especially in children. Helps with bronchitis and emphysema and also helps clear copious catarrh.

False unicorn root
Chamaelirium luteum One of the best tonics for the female reproductive system. Take as a decoction, half-cup, twice daily, or as a tincture, 15 drops, twice daily. **Caution:** *Do not exceed the dose as large amounts may cause nausea or vomiting. Do not take in pregnancy.*

Fennel
Foeniculum vulgare Excellent remedy for colic and flatulence. Helps increase milk flow in breastfeeding.

Forskolin
Coleus forskohlii Used to aid digestion, help reduce blood pressure, and improve circulation.

Golden rod
Solidago virgaurea Helpful for coughs, colds, and sinusitis. Useful for clearing catarrh in acute and chronic cases.

Horsetail
Equisetum arvense Diuretic and astringent helpful in the treatment of urinary disorders, including bedwetting and incontinence.

Hyssop

Hyssopus officinalis Helps relieve coughs and colds. Also relaxant for anxiety and hysteria.

Juniper berries

Juniperus communis Excellent remedy for cystitis. Also used externally as oil to ease painful muscles and joints. **Caution:** *Do not take in pregnancy or with kidney disease.*

Milk thistle

Silybum marianum Aid to the liver, helping to promote the flow of bile. Excellent remedy to promote milk flow when breastfeeding.

Myrrh

Commiphora molmol Strong anti-microbial action used for the treatment of infections, particularly as mouthwash.

Pilewort

Ranunculus ficaria Used specifically to treat hemorrhoids or piles. Use internally as a tea, or externally as an ointment.

Poke root

Phytolacca americana Valuable remedy to clear catarrh and cleanse the lymph system. **Caution:** *In large doses poke root acts as a purgative.*

Prickly ash bark and berries

Zanthoxylum americanum Stimulating tonic for the circulatory system. Helpful for many complaints, such as poor circulation, varicose veins, and cramps.

Raspberry leaves

Rubus ideaus Toning for the womb. **Caution:** *Use only during the last three months of pregnancy.*

Red clover

Trifolium pratense Useful remedy for childhood eczema and hyperactivity, helps to cleanse the system.

Slippery elm

Ulmus fulva Soothing herb for digestive complaints. Also used externally as a poultice to treat boils and abscesses. Take as decoction, using one part powder to eight parts water, or as pills.

Stone root

Collinsonia canadensis Mainly used in the treatment of stones or gravel in the urinary system and the gallbladder.

Tea tree

Melaleuca alternifolia Used for its antiseptic and anti-fungal properties. **Caution:** *Can irritate the skin so use in a carrier/base oil for athlete's foot and insect bites.*

Thuja

Thuja occidentalis Used externally to treat warts and fungal infections. **Caution:** *Use internally only under professional supervision.*

Vervain

Verbena officinalis Nervine tonic that will strengthen the nervous system while relaxing and easing tension. Useful for depression following influenza.

Wild oats

Avena sativa Bridge between food and medicine. Useful as general tonic for the nervous system, especially in cases of debility or exhaustion. Anti-depressant. Take as gruel, porridge, or tincture.

Wild yam

Dioscorea villosa Valuable herb that has anti-spasmodic, anti-inflammatory, and anti-rheumatic properties, as well as many properties found in the contraceptive pill. Used for colic, painful periods, and arthritis.

Yellow dock

Rumex crispus Useful for skin complaints and in treating constipation. Promotes the flow of bile, and encourages the action of the gallbladder.

KITCHEN REMEDIES

Basic ingredients found in nearly every kitchen can be used as herbal remedies. Listed below are some common ailments and kitchen remedies which can be used to treat them gently and effectively.

COLDS AND FLU

To make a warming drink, combine 5 ml (1 tsp) lemon juice with one crushed clove of garlic, a tablespoon of honey, and a pinch of either powdered cinnamon or ginger, and pour on a cupful of hot water. The lemon juice is antiseptic and contains vitamin C to fight off a cold; the garlic is antibiotic, helps reduce catarrh, and is good for all kinds of infections; while the cinnamon and ginger are warming.

TOOTHACHE

To ease an aching tooth until you can see a dentist, hold a clove in your mouth over the tooth and slowly nibble away at it. You should not use more than two cloves at any one time, and should not swallow the pieces. If you have the oil, use one or two drops on a small piece of cotton and hold over the tooth to obtain relief. Repeat twice if needed. Cloves are both antiseptic and pain-killing.

ITCHING SKIN/ECZEMA

Ordinary porridge oats can be used to alleviate itching skin and heal eczema. Prepare a decoction of the oats, strain, and add the liquid to a lukewarm bath (*see* Herbal Methods section). Externally, oats are soothing and healing to the skin as well as cleansing. Taken as porridge or as a juice, oats are nutritious and strengthen the nervous system, acting as an antidepressant, and also helping to reduce cholesterol.

COUGHS AND SORE THROATS

Take half an onion, sliced, and alternate the layers with sugar on a plate. Place a bowl over this and leave overnight before pouring off the juice, which makes an excellent cough syrup. Onions are both antiseptic and healing.

DIARRHEA

A simple but effective emergency treatment is to drink a cup of ordinary tea without milk or sugar. The tannins will coat the lining of the stomach and astringe it, relieving the symptoms. For children, dilute fresh lemon juice with water and add a little honey. If this condition persists you must seek additional help as you run the risk of dehydrating, which is potentially very serious.

STINGS AND BITES

To alleviate the pain from insect stings and bites use cold cider vinegar as a wash. To prevent insect bites, especially before going away on vacation, eat plenty of garlic, as it will dissuade insects from bothering you.

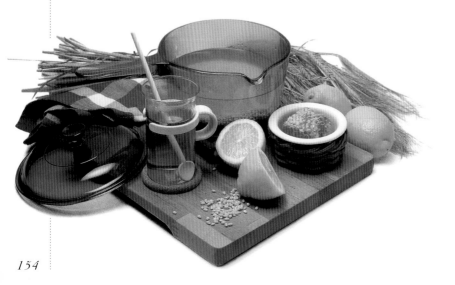

A FAMILY REMEDY CHEST

A home herbal medicine chest can be prepared in addition to a conventional first-aid kit, but should not replace it. (A conventional kit will contain such necessities as bandages, scissors, and thermometer.) The essentials can be supplemented by a range of herbal remedies which will enhance your family's well-being.

OBTAINING YOUR REMEDIES

Some of the remedies will be available commercially. Others may be obtained by using the Herbal Methods section (see pp.14–31) to prepare the ointments, creams, etc. which will be useful for you and your family. Refer to the Herbal Directory (see pp. 100–151) for information on individual herbs and their dosages, or refer to the general dosages information in the Herbal Methods section (see p.16). Commercial remedies will state recommended dosage.

PILLS

SLIPPERY ELM
A useful remedy which will ease diarrhea and gastric upsets. Also available as a powder.

ECHINACEA
Invaluable for infections; antiviral and antibacterial.

CAPSULES

GARLIC OIL
Use to combat infections. Take before and during a vacation to deter insect bites. For ear infections, open capsule, place two drops on a small piece of cotton, and place in ear.

CREAMS

ARNICA
Use for bruises and sprains. Do not apply to broken skin. Discontinue when discoloration disappears.

COMFREY
Use on skin area over sprains, strains, and fractures. Do not apply to broken skin.

OINTMENTS

CALENDULA
Use for cuts and grazes. Ideal for children, and may be used for diaper rash to protect baby's skin.

ESSENTIAL OILS

LAVENDER
Apply to mild burns after cooling for 10 minutes. Acts as pain-killer. Use neat on insect bites and stings. See Herbal Directory for its many other uses (see p.125).

THYME
Use as inhalation (see Herbal Methods, p.24) to ease breathing, catarrh, or sinusitis. Add five drops to a bath to relieve tired and aching muscles.

GEL

ALOE VERA
Use gel or keep the fresh plant on hand and break a leaf off when needed. Heals cuts and scrapes. Good for sunburn and itchy skin.

HERBS

Which herbs you keep on hand will be entirely a matter of personal choice. However, some suggestions might be, camomile to calm digestive upsets and aid sleep; elderflower for colds and flu, hayfever, etc.; limeblossom for poor sleep and shock; meadowsweet for an acid stomach, arthritic pains, and headaches; nettle for allergies and heavy bleeding.

GLOSSARY

A brief description of some of the terms used in this book.

Alterative
Acts as a blood cleanser.

Anodyne
Pain killer.

Antiallergenic
Helps reduce allergic reactions.

Antibacterial
Works against bacteria which cause infection.

Anticarcinogenic
Works against cancer.

Anticatarrhal
Reduces excess catarrh.

Anticholesterol
Reduces cholesterol levels.

Antidepressant
Active against depression.

Antiemetic
Helps prevent vomiting.

Antifungal
Works against fungal infections.

Antihemorrhagic
Helps prevent bleeding.

Anti-inflammatory
Reduces inflammation.

Antioxidant
Helps prevent breakdown of tissues.

Antispasmodic
Reduces muscle spasm.

Antithrombotic
Reduces blood clotting levels.

Antiviral
Works against viruses which cause infection.

Antiseptic
Helps prevent infection.

Astringent
Coats the surface of the skin, reducing fluids and bleeding.

Carminative
Helps relieve indigestion.

Counterirritant
Causes local irritation by drawing blood thus acting as pain-reliever.

Decongestant
Eases congestion caused by excess mucus.

Demulcent
Coats surface, soothing and aiding healing.

Diaphoretic
Encourages removal of toxins through sweating.

Diuretic
Helps relieve water retention by encouraging urination.

Edema
Swelling of the tissues due to excess water retention.

Emmenagogue
Encourages menstruation by stimulating uterine muscles.

Emollient
Soothing to the skin.

Expectorant
Promotes cough reflex, aiding the expulsion of phlegm.

Exudate
Discharge from sore or wound.

Hemostatic
Reduces bleeding.

Hyperthyroid
Over-activity of the thyroid gland.

Hypoglycemic
Reduces blood sugar levels.

Laxative
Promotes mild bowel evacuation.

Mucilage
Gelatinous, demulcent, and soothing.

Neuralgia
Nerve pain or irritation.

Purgative
Promotes strong evacuation of the bowels.

Refrigerant
Cooling and pain-relieving.

Relaxant
Relaxes muscles.

Sedative
Reduces activity of the nervous system.

Soporific
Causes drowsiness or sleep.

Tonic
Re-balances and nourishes the system.

Topically
External use.

Vulnary
Wound-healer.

FURTHER READING AND USEFUL ADDRESSES

Books and journals
Bensky, D. and Barlott, R., *Chinese Herbal Medicine—Formulas and Strategies*. Eastland Press. Washington D.C., 1990.

Chevallier, A., *The Encyclopedia of Medicinal Plants*. Dorling Kindersley. London, 1996.

Fratkin, J., *Herbal Patent Formulas: A Practical Guide*. Institute for Traditional Medicine. Portland, Oregon, 1986.

Grieve, M., *A Modern Herbal*. Penguin Books. London, 1989.

Hoffman, D., *The Holistic Herbal*. Element Books. Dorset, 1983.

Lust, J., *The Herb Book*. Bantam. New York, 1986.

McIntyre, A., *The Herbal for Mother and Child*. Element Books. Dorset, 1992.

McIntyre, A., *Herbs for Common Ailments*. Gaia Books. London, 1992.

Ody, P., *The Complete Medicinal Herbal*. Dorling Kindersley. London, 1993.

Vogel, V., *American Indian Medicine*. University of Oklahoma Press, 1970.

Wren, R. C., *Potter's New Cyclopaedia of Botanical Drugs and Preparations*. C. W. Daniel Company Ltd. Saffron Walden, Essex, 1988.

The Canadian Journal of Herbalism. 11 Winthrop Place, Stoney Creek, Ontario, L8G 3M3, Canada.

European Journal of Herbal Medicine. National Institute of Medical Herbalists, 56 Longbrook Street, Exeter, Devon EX4 6AH, England.

Where to find a qualified practitioner
The National Institute of Medical Herbalists (est. 1864), 56 Longbrook Street, Exeter, Devon EX4 6AH, England.

The General Council and Register of Consultant Herbalists, 18 Sussex Square, Brighton, East Sussex BN2 5AA, England.

Ontario Herbalists Association, 7 Alpine Avenue, Toronto, Ontario M6P 3R6, Canada.

American Holistic Medical Association, 6728 Old McLean Village Drive, McLean, VA 22101–3906, USA.

American Herbalist Guild, PO Box 1683, Soquel, CA 95073, USA.

National Herbalists Association of Australia, Suite 305, BST House, 3 Smail Street, Broadway, NSW 2007, Australia.

Courses
Middlesex University, Queensway, Enfield, Middlesex EN3 4SF, England. Full-time and correspondence courses.

Australasian College of Natural Therapies, 56 Foveaux Street, PO Box K1356, Haymarket 1240, Surry Hills, NSW 2012, Australia.

Australian College of Natural Medicine, 362 Water Street, Fortitude Valley, QLD 4007, Australia.

Southern School of Natural Therapies, 43 Victoria Street, Fitzroy, VIC 3065, Australia.

SA College of Natural Therapies and Traditional Chinese Medicine, 307–309 Pulteney Street, Adelaide, SA 5000, Australia.

The Dominion Herbal College (est. 1926), 7527 Kingsway, Burnaby, British Columbia V3N 3C1, Canada. Correspondence courses only.

The Canadian School of Phytotherapy (Herbal Medicine), Mohawk College, Hamilton, Ontario, Canada.

National College of Naturopathic Medicine, 11231 S. E. Market St, Portland, OR 97216, USA.

INDEX

abscesses 50–1, 73–4
acne 73, 74
adrenal glands 44, 54, 67, 69
aerobic exercise 41, 78
agrimony 57
AIDS 10
alcohol 34
allergies 33
aloe vera 105, 155
anemia 83
angelica 9, 33, 34, 35, 62, 107
Angelica and Loranthus Pill
  (*Du Huo Ji Sheng Wan*) 34,
  87
antiseptics 21
anxiety 18, 91-2
arnica 152, 155
  tincture (recipe) 75, 87
aromatherapy 90
arteriosclerosis 79–80
arthritis 34, 39, 85–6
asthma 35, 40, 44–5, 70
astragalus 9, 34, 62, 110
athlete's foot 74
atractylodis 33, 35

Ba Zhen Wan 33, 60
backache/pain 34, 35, 87
barberry 61
barley water 55–6
baths 23, 82
bedwetting 57
belching 50
Bi Yan Pian 33–4, 45
Bible 8
bilberry 47
bites 30, 154
bladder 54
bladderwrack 69, 152
blepharitis 46
bloating 34, 35, 50, 52, 53
blood, nourishing 34, 35
blood pressure:
  high 34, 80–1
  low 81
blood sugar 67–8
boils 30, 73–4
boneset 12, 43, 152
borage 62, 69, 152
breastfeeding 62–3
breasts, painful 63
breathing process 40
Bright Eyes Rehmannia Pills
  (*Ming Mu Di Huang Wan*)
  35, 47
bronchitis 35

bruises 75
Bu Zhong Yi Qi Wan 34, 52, 56
bugleweed 152
burdock 35, 108
burns 75

cabbage leaves 63, 74
caffeine 56, 90–1
calendula (pot marigold) 21,
  22, 26, 111, 155
camomile 12, 19, 22, 27,
  112, 155
cancer 10, 40
caraway 8
cardamom 50
caster oil 8
cataracts 46–7
catarrh 24, 43
catnip 152
cayenne 81, 82, 152
celery seed 152
Central *Qi* Pills (*Bu Zhong Yi
  Qi Wan*) 34, 52, 56
chaste berry 149
chest infections 44
Chesty cough remedy
  (recipe) 20
chicken livers 57
chickweed 27, 138
chilblains 82
childbirth 33, 62
chilli 82
Chinese herbalism 9
  herbal decoctions 32
  patent formulas 33–5
Chinese herbals 8
Chinese medicine 41
chiropractic 94–5
cholesterol 77, 80
Christianity 8–9
chrysanthemum 33, 35, 113
cinnamon 34, 43, 81, 82,
  152, 154
circulation 33, 34, 35, 82–3
circulatory system 76–9
citrus peel 34
Clear Air Tea (*Qi Hua Tan
  Wan*) 35, 45
cleavers 120
clover 153
cloves 50, 82, 152, 154
codonopsis 34, 35
Codonopsis, Piroa,
  Atractylodes Formula
  (Shen *Ling Bai Zhu Pian*)
  35, 50

cohosh, black 114
Cold and flu tea (recipe) 17
cold sores 74
colds 12, 24, 35, 39, 42, 154
colic 50
coltsfoot 145
comfrey 139, 155
compresses 30
conceiving, difficulty in 65
congestion 24
conjunctivitis 22, 46
constipation 48, 49–50
contraceptive pill, stopping
  61
coriander 8
cornsilk 150
couchgrass 55, 56, 57
Cough syrup (recipe) 28
coughs 20, 28, 35, 44, 154
counseling 90
crampbark 148
cranberry 55
creams 27
cuts and scrapes 26
cystitis 55–6

damiana 69, 152
dandelion 142
dandruff 74
Dang Gui Si Ni Tang
  (Decoction for Frigid
  Extremities) 34, 83
decoctions 18, 32
depression 92
devil's claw 86
diabetes 67–8
diarrhea 48, 50, 52–3, 154
diet 11
diet supplements 60
diffusers 24
digestion, strengthening 34,
  35
digestive complaints 11
digestive system 48–9
Dioscorides 8
dizziness 33, 35
dock, yellow 83, 133
dosage 16
drawing paste (recipe) 30
drugs, combining with herbs
  39
Dry-scalp rinse (recipe) 29
drying herbs 15
Du Huo Ji Sheng Wan 34, 87
duodenal ulcers 48, 52
dustmites 44

ear ailments 46, 47
Ear-ringing Left Loving Pills
  (*Er Long Zuo Ci Wan*) 34
earache 47
echinacea 12, 116, 155
eczema 70, 72, 74, 154
Egyptians 8
elderflower 17, 29, 135, 155
elecampane 20, 152
emphysema 40
endocrine system 66–7
endometriosis 61
environment, herbs and
  10–12
Er Long Zuo Ci Wan 34
essential oils 39
eucalyptus 24, 43
evening primrose 60, 65, 86
exercise 11, 41, 78, 90
extremities, warming 34
eyebaths 22, 46
eyebright 22, 118
eyes 22, 34, 35, 46–7
eyewashes 22

false unicorn root 152
fennel 152
fever 35, 42
feverfew 140
flatulence 51, 52
flu *see* influenza
folk medicine 9
food poisoning 50
foot bath 23, 82
forskolin 152
forsythia 34, 35, 42
Four Gentlemen Decoction
  (*Si Jun Zi Tang*) 33
frankincense 64
Free and Easy Wanderer
  (*Xiao Yao Wan*) 35, 53, 60
frostbite 34
fungal infections 74–5

Galen 8
gallbladder 53
gargles 21
garlic 8, 12, 29, 47, 97, 104,
  155
gastric ulcer 51–2
gastritis 51
geranium 63, 64
ginger 12, 20, 23, 34, 43,
  151, 154
gingivitis 50
ginkgo 121

ginseng 9, 32, 33, 91, 117
Ginseng Medicinal Brandy
  (recipe) 65
glaucoma 46–7
glossary 156–7
glue ear 46, 47
golden rod 152
goldenseal 123
gout 86
Greeks 8
guelder rose see crampbark

hand bath 23, 82
hawthorn 39, 115
hayfever 33, 40, 45
headaches 11, 34, 35, 94
healing herbs 38–9
heartburn 51
Heavenly King Benefit
  Heart Pill (Tian Wang Bu
  Xin Wan) 35, 93
hemorrhoids 31, 34, 53
herbalism, history 8–9
herbalists 39
herbals 8
herbs:
  buying 15
  cautions and
    contraindications 38–9
  combining 9
  combining with drugs 39
  dosage 16
  drying 15
  and environment 10–12
  growing 15
  obtaining 14–15
  parts to use 14–15
  picking 14–15
  storing 15
  substances in 9
  uses 11–12
  using safely 12
herpes simplex 74
Hippocrates 8
hives 73
holistic health 10–12
honeycomb 45
honeysuckle 35, 42, 127
hops 9, 92, 93, 95
hormones 66, 67, 68
horsetail 152
hot flushes 63
hyperactivity 93–4
hypertension see blood
  pressure, high
hyssop 153

immune system 34, 44, 96–7
immunity, low 11
impotence 64
incontinence 56–7
indigestion 19, 35, 50, 51
infertility 64
influenza 12, 17, 24, 35, 39,
  43, 154
infused oils 25
infusions 17

inhalations 24, 43
insect bites and stings 30, 154
insomnia 34, 35, 92–3
intestines 52
Iron tonic recipe 20
irritability 35
irritable bowel syndrome
  (IBS) 52–3
itching 154
Itchy-skin lotion (recipe) 29

jasmine 64
joint pains 64
juniper 83, 153

kelp 65, 69
kidneys 35, 54–5
  infections 57
  stones 57
kitchen remedies 154

labor 62
lady's mantle 103
laurel 8
lavender 12, 24, 26, 30, 61,
  125, 155
lemon 82, 154
lemon balm 129
licorice 33, 34, 64, 83, 86,
  122
life force 10–11
limeblossom (flower) 144,
  155
linseed 49, 56
Liu Wei Di Huang Wan 35,
  47, 87
liver 35, 53, 96
Lonicera, Forsythia Dispel
  Heat Tablets (Yin Qiao Jie
  Du Pian) 35, 42
lungs 40–1
Lycium, Chrysanthemum,
  Rehmannia Pills (Qi Ju Di
  Huang Wan) 35, 47
lycium fruit 9, 35, 64, 86,
  128
lymphatic system 96

macular degeneration 46–7
maize 150
male fern 61
marigold see calendula
marshmallow 30, 106
massage 90
mastitis 63
meadowsweet 119, 155
medicine chest 155
meditation 11, 41, 90
menopause 35, 63
menstrual cycle 58
menstrual disorders 33, 35,
  59, 60–1
mental agitation 35
migraines 50, 94–5
milk thistle 153
Ming Mu Di Huang Wan 35,
  47

mint 8
miscarriage, threatened
  61–2
monasteries 9
morning sickness 50, 62
Morus, Chrysanthemum
  Medicine Pill (Sang Ju Yin
  Pian) 35, 45
motherwort 60, 126
mouth abscesses 50–1
mouth problems 50–1
mouth ulcers 21, 50, 51
mouth-freshening recipe 21
mouthwashes 21
moxa 60, 87
mugwort 60, 87, 109
muscular stiffness 35
musculoskeletal system 84–5
mustard 23
myrrh 21, 74, 153

nausea 50
neroli 64
nervous exhaustion 95
nervous system 88–91
nervousness 50
nettles 20, 146, 155
neuralgia 95
nicotine 90
Nose Inflammation Pills (Bi
  Yan Pian) 33–4, 45

oats 153, 154
oil infusions 25
ointments 26
onions 154
opium 8
osteopathy 94–5

palpitations 35, 79
pancreas 67–8
pao d'arco 141
parsley 60
passion flower (passiflora) 9,
  131
patent formulas, Chinese
  33–5
pennyroyal 61
peppermint 12, 17, 23, 35,
  42, 130
perilla leaf 62
pessaries 31
pilewort 153
pine needles 43
poke root 153
pollution 41
poria 33, 35
porridge oats 154
pot marigold see calendula
poultices 30, 74
pregnancy 61
  herbs to avoid 61
  precautions during 38–9
premenstrual tension (PMT)
  60
preventative treatment 12
prickly ash 82, 153

prostatitis 56
psoriasis 73
psychotherapy 90
psyllium seeds 49
pumpkin seeds 56
purple cone flower see
  echinacea

qi 9, 41
Qi Hua Tan Wan 35, 45
Qi Ju Di Huang Wan 35, 47

raspberry leaf 62, 153
Raynaud's disease 34, 83
rectum, prolapses 34
relaxation 11, 90
reproductive system 58–9
respiration 40–2
respiratory disease,
  prevention 41
restlessness 35
rheumatism 85–6
rhubarb leaves 63
Romans 8
rose 64, 65, 80, 92, 93
rosehip 12
rosemary 61, 132
royal jelly 65
rue 153

safflower 56
sage 21, 134
St John's wort 25, 124
Salad dressing (recipe) 29
salt compress 87
Sang Ju Yin Pian 35, 45
saw palmetto 137
scalp 29
sciatica 34, 87, 95
seasonal adjustment disorder
  (SAD) 92
sex drive, low, in women 64
shen 35
Shen Ling Bai Zhu Pian 35, 50
shingles 95
Si Jun Zi Tang 33
sinus infections 35, 43–4
sinusitis 24
Six-flavor Rehmannia Pill
  (Liu Wei Di Huang Wan)
  35, 47, 87
skin 27, 29, 70–2
skin disease, preventing 71
skullcap 18, 136
sleep, inducing 9
sleep-pillows 93
sleeplessness see insomnia
slippery elm 30, 153, 155
smoking 40–1, 77
sneezing 35
Soothing cream (recipe) 27
sore throats 35, 43, 154
sperm count, low 65
spirituality 11
spleen 35
splinters 30
sprains 87

squaw vine 62
steam inhalation 43
steroids 69, 152
stiffness, easing 34
stings 30, 154
stomach 51–2
stone root 153
stools, problems 35, 50, 52
storage of herbs 15
stress 11, 52, 78–9, 91
Stress and anxiety drink (recipe) 18
styes 46
Suan Zao Ren Tang Pian 35, 93
Sumerians 8
suppositories 31
syrups 28

tachycardia 79
t'ai chi 11

tansy 61
tea 154
tea tree 153
teas (infusions) 12, 17
tension 24, 52
thirst 34
thuja 61, 153
thyme 8, 24, 28, 143, 155
thyroid 35, 67, 68–9
Tian Wang Bu Xin Wan 35, 93
tinctures 19
tinnitus 34, 35, 46, 47
Tired eyes remedy (recipe) 22
tiredness 33
tisanes (infusions) 17
tonics 20, 35, 53
tonsillitis 43
tonsils 43
toothache 50, 154

ulcers:
  duodenal 48, 52
  gastric 51–2
  mouth 50
urethritis 55–6
urinary system 54
urticaria 73
uterus, prolapses 34

valerian 9, 18, 147
vaporizers 24
varicose veins 34, 82
verbena 18, 92
vervain 153
vinegars 29
vomiting 50

warts 74
water retention 56
Western herbalism 9
wild oats 153

wild yam 153
willow bark 95
wines, medicinal 20
witch hazel 31, 63, 75, 82
Women's Precious Pills (*Ba Zhen Wan*) 33, 60
wormwood 61
wounds 75

Xiao Yao Wan 35, 53, 60

yam 153
yarrow 17, 42, 102
Yin Qiao Jie Du Pian 35, 42
yin and *yang* 9
yoga 11, 41

Zyziphys Seed Soup Tablet (*Suan Zao Ren Tang Pian*) 35, 93

CREDITS

Quarto would like to acknowledge and thank the following for providing pictures used in this in this book. While every effort has been made to acknowledge copyright holders we would like to apologize should there have been any omissions.

Key: *t*=top *b*=bottom *c*=center *l*=left *r*=right

Pat Brindley p.104, p.109, p.112, p.116, p.125, p.127, p.130, p.132, p.134; **Julian Cotton** p.69(*b*); **Harry Smith Horticultural Photographic Collection** p.102, p.103, p.105, p.106, p.108, p.110, p.111, p.113, p.115, p.118, p.122, p.124, p.128, p.129, p.133, p.135, p.136, p.138, p.140, p.141, p.142, p.143, p.144, p.145, p.146, p.147, p.148, p.149, p.150, p.151; **The Image Bank** p.24, p.41(*c*), p.52(*b*), p.53(*t*), p.57(*b*), p.62(*b*), p.68(*t*), p.73(*t*), p.75(*t*); **Peter McHoy** p.107, p.114, p.119, p.120, p.121, p.139; **Photos Horticultural Picture Library** p.126; **Photo/Nats Inc.** p.123, p.131, p.137; **Positive Images** p.117; **Pictor International** p.16, p.26, p.39(*tr*), p.61(*b*), p.64(*b*), p.72(*t*), p.78(*b*), p.80(*b*), p.87(*b*), p.95(*t*), p.98(*t*); **Tony Stone Images** p.9, p.11, p.27, p.28, p.41(*b*), p.42(*t*), p.45(*b*), p.47(*b*), p.51(*t*), p.56(*t*), p.63(*t*), p.74(*b*), p.78(*t*), p.79(*t*), p.83(*t*), p.86(*t*), p.90(*l*), p.91(*b*), p.92(*t*), p.93(*b*).

All other photographs are the copyright of Quarto.
Quarto would also like to thank the following for supplying props and equipment for photography:

Plasterworks 38 Cross Street, London N1 2BG.

Neal's Yard Remedies Neal's Yard, Covent Garden, London WC2.

East West Herbs Ltd. 3 Neal's Yard, London WC2.

Authors' acknowledgments
This book is dedicated with my dearest love and thanks to Mary for her support, Kelly for her encouragement, and to Megan, who gives me joy and inspiration. **Jade Britton**

To Clive, Ryan and Molly Jo, with thanks for your love and support, and to my beautiful garden. **Tamara Kircher**

Senior Art Editor: **Elizabeth Healey**
Editor: **Judith Evans**
Designer: **Caroline Hill**
Photographer: **Bruce Mackie**
Illustrator: **Kevin Maddison**
Picture Researcher: **Zoë Holtermann**
Indexer: **Dorothy Frame**
Managing Editor: **Sally MacEachern**
Editorial Director: **Pippa Rubinstein**
Assistant Art Director: **Penny Cobb**
Art Director: **Moira Clinch**